Chronic Myeloid Leukemia

Chronic Myeloid Leukemia

Edited by

Jorge Cortes

*University of Texas M.D. Anderson Cancer Center
Houston, Texas, U.S.A.*

Michael Deininger

*Oregon Health & Science University
Portland, Oregon, U.S.A.*

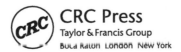

CRC Press
Taylor & Francis Group
Boca Raton London New York

CRC Press is an imprint of the
Taylor & Francis Group, an **informa** business

First published 2007 by Informa Healthcare, Inc.

Published 2019 by CRC Press
Taylor & Francis Group
6000 Broken Sound Parkway NW, Suite 300
Boca Raton, FL 33487-2742

First issued in paperback 2019

No claim to original U.S. Government works

ISBN 13: 978-0-367-45330-5 (pbk)
ISBN 13: 978-0-8493-7955-0 (hbk)

**Visit the Taylor & Francis Web site at
http://www.taylorandfrancis.com**

**and the CRC Press Web site at
http://www.crcpress.com**

Preface

Chronic myeloid leukemia (CML) is a rare disease and yet it has had a profound impact on the development of modern, evidence-based medicine. Some 160 years ago the term leukemia was coined when Bennet, and almost simultaneously Virchov, described the striking white appearance of the blood of two patients with, presumably, CML. The discovery of the Philadelphia chromosome (Ph), first described as a minute chromosome 22 by Nowel and Hungerford in 1960, marks the first consistent association between a chromosomal abnormality and a specific malignancy, proving that alterations of DNA are causal to cancer. Thirteen years later it was Janet Rowley who recognized that Ph is in fact the result of a chromosomal translocation involving chromosomes 9 and 22. A decade later Bartram and Groffen identified the genes juxtaposed by the t(9;22) as ABL and BCR. Shortly thereafter the central role of tyrosine kinase activity for Bcr-Abl's ability to induce malignant transformation was recognized and murine models developed by Daley and colleagues generated experimental evidence that Bcr-Abl is necessary and probably sufficient to induce the chronic phase of CML. This provided a rationale for using pharmacological inhibitors of Bcr-Abl for the treatment of CML and ultimately led to the clinical development of imatinib by Druker and colleagues.

Imatinib has completely changed the CML landscape. Ten years ago there were few therapeutic choices. Allogeneic stem cell transplant was recommended to patients with a suitable donor and deemed fit to undergo the procedure. All other patients were treated with an interferon-alpha-based regimen, realizing that only a minority would achieve durable responses and become long-term survivors. This is history: the rate of complete cytogenetic response in newly diagnosed patients treated with imatinib approaches 90%, with many patients attaining more than 1000-fold reductions of their leukemia burden as measured by polymerase chain reaction (PCR). With the revolution of therapy came fundamental changes in monitoring. Quantitative PCR to measure the level of BCR-ABL transcripts, previously relevant only in the setting of allogeneic transplant, has become key to monitoring the majority of patients once they have achieved a complete cytogenetic response. For many CML patients the perception of their disease has evolved from being a deadly illness worth accepting the risks of an allogeneic transplant to becoming a chronic ailment that can be controlled for long periods of time with an oral medication that causes little if any discomfort. Despite the impressive responses achieved with imatinib in most patients, resistance develops in some patients with early disease and is frequent in those who start treatment in accelerated phase or blast crisis. Point mutations in the kinase domain of Bcr-Abl have been identified as the leading known mechanism of resistance to imatinib, again generating a novel paradigm in oncology. The problem of clinical resistance has led to the development of novel, more potent Bcr-Abl inhibitors that maintain activity against mutant Bcr-Abl and may eventually prove superior to imatinib as first-line therapy.

With all this, the management of CML has become a complex undertaking. While prescribing the pills is seemingly easy, exploiting the full potential of the novel therapies requires considerable knowledge and skills. The rapid accumulation of new data makes it ever harder to stay on top of this rapidly evolving field, even for CML experts. This defines the purpose of this book: to provide rapid, easy access to the most recent information. A panel of leaders in the field has been assembled to provide a comprehensive and yet condensed overview of CML in the year 2006, covering the most topical aspects of CML biology, diagnostics, therapy and monitoring. To do this we aimed at a very short lag period between conception of the book, writing of the chapters and publication of the final product to keep the information as current as possible. In a field as rapidly evolving as this, it is inevitable that new information will be available by the time this book reaches the reader. But we are confident that this formidable effort will still provide very current and valid information. We hope that the reader will find this book a useful guide to stay current in a complex field.

Jorge Cortes
Michael Deininger

Contents

Contributors

Mukta Arora Department of Hematology, Oncology and Transplantation, University of Minnesota, Minneapolis, Minnesota, U.S.A.

David J. Barnes Department of Haematology, Imperial College London, Hammersmith Hospital, London, U.K.

Monica Bocchia Department of Hematology, Siena University, Siena, Italy

Susan Branford Institute of Medical and Veterinary Science, Adelaide, South Australia

Bruno Calabretta Department of Microbiology and Immunology, Kimmel Cancer Center, Thomas Jefferson Medical College, Philadelphia, Pennsylvania, U.S.A.

Jorge Cortes Department of Leukemia, University of Texas M.D. Anderson Cancer Center, Houston, Texas, U.S.A.

Michael Deininger Oregon Health & Science University, Portland, Oregon, U.S.A.

Justus Duyster Department of Internal Medicine III, Klinikum rechts der Isar, Technical University of Munich, Munich, Germany

Francis Giles Department of Leukemia, University of Texas M.D. Anderson Cancer Center, Houston, Texas, U.S.A.

John M. Goldman Hematology Branch, National Institutes of Health, Bethesda, Maryland, U.S.A.

François Guilhot Department of Oncology-Hematology and Cell Therapy, Clinical Research Centre, Poitiers, France

Mary M. Horowitz Department of Medicine, Centre for International Blood and Marrow Transplant Research, Medical College of Wisconsin, Milwaukee, Wisconsin, U.S.A.

Timothy P. Hughes Institute of Medical and Veterinary Science, Adelaide, South Australia

Nicola Hurst Institute of Medical and Veterinary Science, Adelaide, South Australia

Elias Jabhour Department of Leukemia, University of Texas M.D. Anderson Cancer Center, Houston, Texas, U.S.A.

Hagop Kantarjian Department of Leukemia, University of Texas M.D. Anderson Cancer Center, Houston, Texas, U.S.A.

Francesco Lauria Department of Hematology, Siena University, Siena, Italy

Géraldine Martineau Department of Oncology-Hematology and Cell Therapy, Clinical Research Centre, Poitiers, France

Junia V. Melo Department of Haematology, Imperial College London, Hammersmith Hospital, London, U.K.

Frédéric Millot Department of Oncology-Hematology and Cell Therapy, Clinical Research Centre, Poitiers, France

Susan O'Brien Department of Leukemia, University of Texas M.D. Anderson Cancer Center, Houston, Texas, U.S.A.

Danilo Perrotti Human Cancer Genetics Program, Department of Molecular Virology, Immunology and Medical Genetics and the Comprehensive Cancer Center, The Ohio State University, Columbus, Ohio, U.S.A.

Alfonso Quintás-Cardama Department of Leukemia, University of Texas M.D. Anderson Cancer Center, Houston, Texas, U.S.A.

Lydia Roy Department of Oncology-Hematology and Cell Therapy, Clinical Research Centre, Poitiers, France

Nikolas von Bubnoff Department of Internal Medicine III, Klinikum rechts der Isar, Technical University of Munich, Munich, Germany

BCR-ABL as a Molecular Target

Michael Deininger
Oregon Health & Science University, Portland, Oregon, U.S.A.

INTRODUCTION

BCR-ABL, the product of the t(9;22)(q34;q11), is cytogenetically apparent as the Philadelphia chromosome (Ph) and is critical to the pathogenesis of chronic myeloid leukemia (CML). It occurs in approximately 25% of patients with acute lymphoblastic leukemia (ALL). In CML, the presence of *BCR-ABL* defines the disease; in ALL it defines a subset of patients with a very poor prognosis. *BCR-ABL* is a constitutively active tyrosine kinase, a feature that is critical to the protein's ability to induce leukemia and provides the rational basis for Abl kinase targeted therapy of Ph-positive leukemias with Abl kinase inhibitors. This chapter will focus on *BCR-ABL* as target for the therapy of CML.

CLINICAL FEATURES OF CHRONIC MYELOID LEUKEMIA

CML has an annual incidence of approximately $1.5/10^5$, accounting for some 5000 new patients per year in the United States. Males are slightly more frequently affected than females (ratio 1.7 : 1), but there is no significant ethnic or geographical predisposition (1). The disease can occur at every age but the incidence greatly increases in the older population. Exposure to ionizing radiation is the only established risk factor, as demonstrated by the increased incidence in the survivors of the atomic bombs in Japan (2). Symptoms include weight loss, fever, and abdominal fullness but at least in the developed countries many patients are asymptomatic at diagnosis, when an abnormal routine blood count leads to a diagnostic work up.

The clinical course of CML is two-phased. Most patients (in Western countries, >90%) are diagnosed in the chronic or stable phase, which is characterized by expansion of the myeloid cell compartment, while cellular differentiation and function is largely maintained. After a variable length of time the disease progresses to blast crisis, which resembles an acute leukemia of myeloid (70%), or lymphoid (20%–30%), or undifferentiated phenotype and carries a poor prognosis (3). In the pre-imatinib era, when drug therapy relied on interferon-alpha-based regimens, the median duration of the chronic phase was approximately five years, with few patients surviving longer than ten years.

CHRONIC MYELOID LEUKEMIA AS A PARADIGM IN ONCOLOGY

By comparison with some common malignancies, CML is rare and thus hardly a major general health problem. Nonetheless, the disease has served as a pacemaker in many aspects of cancer biology and therapy. CML was the first malignant disorder in which a consistent association with a chromosomal abnormality was demonstrated. Ph, described by Nowell and Hungerford in 1960 (4), was originally thought to represent a shortened chromosome 22 (22q-). Subsequent studies revealed, however, that Ph is the result of a reciprocal translocation between chromosomes 9 and 22 (5). This translocation was shown to fuse sequences of the *ABL* gene from chromosome 9q34 downstream of BCR on chromosome 22q11, generating a chimeric *BCR-ABL* gene, which represented the first demonstration of an oncogenic fusion gene (6,7). Shortly thereafter, the Bcr-Abl protein was shown to exhibit constitutive tyrosine kinase activity that was correlated with cellular transformation, and provided the rationale for the development of specific kinase inhibitors for therapeutic use (8). These efforts eventually led to the discovery of imatinib, the success of which has fundamentally changed the management of CML, while at the same time establishing molecularly targeted therapy as a new paradigm in oncology, with implications much beyond the realm of CML. The direct line, from the presence of a specific causal genetic abnormality *BCR-ABL* to its specific targeted therapy, has led the World Health Organization to define CML as a myeloproliferative disorder with a *BCR-ABL* fusion gene (9), and to refer to the *BCR-ABL*-negative disease as atypical CML (aCML), even in cases that are morphologically indistinguishable. It is likely that this sets off another paradigm, in the sense that the molecular rather than the morphologic or the organ-of-origin based criteria will form the basis of oncological disease classification in the future.

MALIGNANT TRANSFORMATION BY Bcr-Abl
Types of *BCR-ABL* Fusion mRNAs and Proteins

The breakpoints in *BCR* localize to the so-called *b*reakpoint *c*luster *r*egions (*bcr*), a fact that is reflected in the gene's name. Depending on where the breaks occur, variable parts of *BCR* are conserved in the Bcr-Abl fusion protein, leading to proteins of different size. Unlike in *BCR*, the breakpoints in *ABL* are spread over a wide genomic region and may occur anywhere upstream of *ABL* exon Ib, downstream of exon Ia, or between the two alternative first exons (Fig. 1). Due to splicing of the primary mRNA, the *BCR* portion is almost invariably fused to *ABL* exon 2, with rare exceptions (10). Three *bcr*s can be distinguished. Breakpoints in the major *bcr* (M-*bcr*) conserve *BCR* sequences up to exon 13 or 14 (formerly referred to as b2 and b3), which give rise to e13a2 or e14a2 mRNAs and lead to the expression of a 210 kD Bcr-Abl protein (p210$^{Bcr-Abl}$). The latter is found in almost all CML patients and approximately one-third of the ALL patients. Breaks in the minor breakpoint cluster region (m-*bcr*) conserve only *BCR* exon 1, yielding an e1a2 mRNA and smaller 185 kD Bcr-Abl protein (p185$^{Bcr-Abl}$) that is characteristic of ALL and which is only very rarely found in CML (10). A third breakpoint cluster region termed μ-*bcr* is located toward the 3' end of *BCR*. Breaks in this region conserve most *BCR* sequences and lead to expression of an e19a2 *BCR-ABL* mRNA and a 230 kD protein that is associated with chronic neutrophilic leukemia, a rather benign condition (10). Altogether, the preservation of longer Bcr sequences in the Bcr-Abl fusion protein appears to attenuate the disease.

Functional Characteristics of Bcr-Abl (Fig. 2)

Abl (also referred to as Abl-1), the human homologue of the Abelson murine leukemia virus, is a tyrosine kinase involved in multiple cellular processes, including DNA repair, integrin signaling, cell cycle regulation, and signal transduction from cell surface receptors (11). *ABL* knockout mice exhibit increased neonatal lethality and suffer from a number of defects, including skeletal malformations, immune dysfunction as well as an ill-defined wasting syndrome (12,13). Apart from the

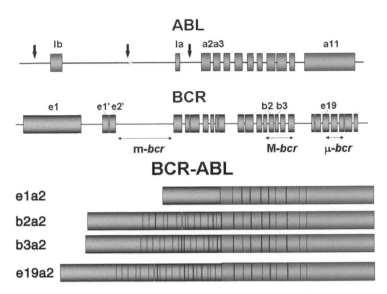

FIGURE 1 Location of the breakpoints in the *ABL* and *BCR* genes and structure of the chimeric mRNAs derived from the various breaks. Note the alternative *ABL* exons Ib and Ia and the large intron between them. Due to splicing of the primary RNA transcript, fusion mRNAs usually contain *ABL* exons a2-a11, regardless of the breakpoint location in *ABL*. In contrast to *ABL*, there is clustering of breakpoints in *BCR*, with three recognized breakpoint cluster regions. Note that the BCR exons b2 and b3 of the old nomenclature are referred to as e13 and e14. With rare exceptions, CML patients have breakpoints in the major breakpoint cluster region (M-*bcr*). The resulting e13a2 and e14a2 fusion mRNAs give rise to a 210kD Bcr-Abl protein.

unique "Cap" region at its very 5' end the N-terminus of Abl has extensive homology to Src kinases (14). The Src homology domains 3 (SH3) and 2 (SH2) mediate interactions with other proteins by binding proline rich regions (SH3) or phosphotyrosine (SH2). The SH1 domain carries the tyrosine kinase function. The large C terminus is unique to Abl and contains DNA binding, nuclear localization, and export signals as well as actin-binding sequences and a proline rich domain(15). In physiological conditions, Abl kinase is tightly regulated by a mechanism that is similar as in Src kinases but uses different structures, as Abl lacks a C-terminal tyrosine that is critical for auto-inhibition of Src kinases (14). In Src, phosphorylation of tyrosine 527 allows the N-terminus to form an intramolecular association with the SH2 domain, inactivating the kinase by forcing the molecule into a "clamp." In Abl, the myristoylated cap binds to a hydrophobic pocket at the base of the kinase domain, resulting in a conformation resembling inactive SRC.

The function of Bcr is largely unknown. The N-terminus of Bcr contains a coiled coil domain that allows for dimerization, which is essential for the transforming capacity of Bcr-Abl and other Abl fusion proteins, such as Etv6-Abl (16). A number of additional structural motifs have been defined, including a serine/threonine kinase activity, guanidine exchange factor (GEF) function, and a GTPase activating function toward small GTPases, including Rac and RhoA. It is thought that the presence of some of these domains in p210$^{Bcr-Abl}$ as opposed to p185$^{Bcr-Abl}$ is responsible for the more benign phenotype of p210$^{Bcr-Abl}$–positive leukemia. Differential activation of Rho family GTPases has been shown in cells expressing

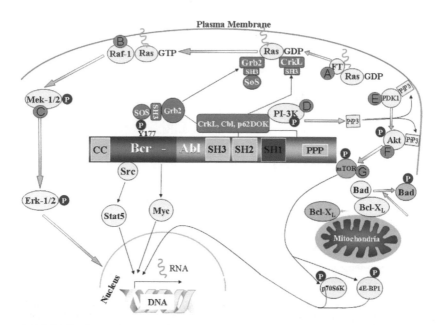

FIGURE 2 Schematic view of signal transduction pathways in cells transformed by Bcr-Abl. Note the SH1 (kinase) domain in Abl, which is absolutely essential for transformation. The coiled coil domain (CC) of Bcr mediates dimerization. SH3, SH2 domains and the proline-rich region (PPP) mediate binding to adaptor proteins including CrkL, Cbl, p62Dok, and others, resulting in the formation of a multiprotein complex. Multiple pathways are activated, including the Ras−mitogen activated protein (MAP) kinase signaling cascade, Phosphatidyl inositol 3′ kinase (PI3′K), Stat5, and Myc. The net effects are inhibition of apoptosis, increased proliferation, perturbed interaction with the bone marrow stroma and genetic instability. Many of the molecules involved are potential drug targets. *(A)* Farnesyl transferases (FT) that prenylate Ras, mediating its binding to the cell membrane, a requirement for activation of Raf; *(B)* Raf, the serine kinase that activates mitogen activated protein (MAP) kinase signaling; *(C)* MAP) kinases; *(D)* phosphatidyl inositol 3′ kinase (PI3′K) that produces 3,4,5 phosphatidyl inositol (PiP$_3$), which is required for localization of Pdk1 and Akt to the inner leaflet of the cell membrane; *(E)* Pdk1 which activates Akt; *(F)* Akt, which activates mammalian target of rapamycin (mTor); *(G)* mTor, which phosphorylates and activates p70S6 kinase and 4E-BP1, two major global regulators of gene transcription in response to growth stimuli. *Source*: From Ref. 51.

p210$^{\text{Bcr-Abl}}$ compared to p185$^{\text{Bcr-Abl}}$, suggesting that they may be important (17). Intriguingly, a recent study suggested that p210$^{\text{Bcr-Abl}}$-positive ALL may arise in a hematopoietic stem cell, in contrast to p185$^{\text{Bcr-Abl}}$-positive disease, which appears to originate in a progenitor cell committed to B-cell differentiation (18). This implies that the two *BCR-ABL* types may have differential capacity to transform hematopoietic stem or progenitor cells, that might be related to their specific abilities to activate critical differentiation specific pathways.

The kinase activity of Bcr-Abl is absolutely required for cellular transformation, implicating it as an excellent therapeutic target. Although there is evidence that effects of Bcr-Abl on some cellular functions (such as migration and adhesion) are kinase-independent, they are currently not thought to be critical to the protein's full leukemogenic potential (19). If nonkinase functions were indeed important, this would obviously limit the efficacy of Bcr-Abl kinase targeted therapy.

Mechanisms of Cellular Transformation by Bcr-Abl (Fig. 2)

Multiple proteins are tyrosine phosphorylated in Bcr-Abl expressing cells, including adaptor proteins such as Shc, cytoskeletal proteins such as paxillin and tensin, transcription factors like Stat5, other kinases including Fes and Hck (a Src kinase), and particularly Bcr-Abl itself (20). Autophosphorylation generates docking sites in Bcr-Abl that allow binding of adaptor proteins such as Grb2 and CrkL that, in turn, recruit additional molecules such as Gab2 and the p85 regulatory subunit of phosphatidyl inositol 3' kinase (PI3K). In some cases, both direct and indirect interactions between Bcr-Abl and the various proteins co-exist (21). The net result is the formation of a multimeric signaling complex that is held together mainly by phosphotyrosine dependent interactions, which implies that Bcr-Abl kinase activity is instrumental to its formation and maintenance. Signaling output from this complex activates multiple pathways, including mitogen activated protein kinases (MAPK) and PI3K/AKT/mTor (22). The result is inhibition of apoptosis, increased proliferation, and a less well-defined perturbation of cellular adhesion to the bone-marrow stroma (15). There is also evidence that Bcr-Abl kinase activity affects DNA repair and induces genomic instability by a variety of mechanisms (23). Defining the precise contribution of various pathways to cellular transformation has been rather difficult. Many early studies have relied on cell lines, which do not adequately reflect the situation in primary cells. More recently, knockout mice have been used to assess the importance of individual components, such as Stat5 (24), IL-3, GM-CSF (25), or Cbl (26). With the exception of Gab2, an adaptor molecule that is crucial to activation of the PI3K pathway and required for induction of myeloid but not lymphoid leukemia (27) and Src kinases, which are required for the induction of B-ALL (28), these studies have been largely negative. This may partially be explained by the fact that the murine CML model, used to determine whether a given protein is crucial, is more aggressive than the rather indolent chronic phase disease in humans. Thus, more subtle differences may be missed. This complex signal transduction network, operated by Bcr-Abl, offers a number of potential drug targets downstream of the initiating lesion, some of which are being evaluated in clinical trials. A comprehensive review of this topic is given in Chapter 9.

Transformation to Blast Crisis

One could argue that chronic phase CML would not pose a significant clinical problem, if it did not lead to blastic transformation. Thus, prevention of blast crisis could be defined as the primary therapeutic goal in CML. The mechanisms responsible for disease progression in CML are currently not well understood. It is conceivable that with more insights into the molecular events that lead to blast crisis, it may be possible to design therapeutic strategies to prevent transformation or reverse blast crisis to chronic phase. The biology of blast crisis is the topic of Chapter 10.

DEVELOPMENT AND PRECLINICAL EVALUATION OF IMATINIB

Starting in the late 1980s, scientists at Ciba Geigy (now Novartis) initiated projects on the identification of compounds with inhibitory activity against protein kinases. One medicinal chemistry project focused on protein kinase C, which at the time was thought to be critical to the pathogenesis of various malignant tumors. This project led to the identification of a 2-phenylaminopyrimidine derivative as the lead compound. The lead compound had low potency and poor specificity, inhibiting tyrosine and serine/threonine kinases with equal potency, but served as the starting point for the synthesis of a number of derivatives. Specific substitutions reduced activity against serine/threonine kinases, increased activity against tyrosine kinases, and improved intracellular activity and water solubility. The end result of these efforts was a compound initially termed CGP57148, then STI571, and eventually imatinib mesylate (Glivec®, Gleevec™).

Imatinib inhibits the kinase activity of Abl- and Abl-derived fusion kinases with an IC_{50} of approximately 25 nM in cell-free assays and 250 nM in cells. Although there are some "off target" activities against the platelet derived growth factor receptor (Pdgfr), Kit, and to a slightly lesser degree Lck, a Src kinase, and Fms (Csfr-1), the overall specificity of imatinib is quite exceptional and unexpected, given the extensive sequence homology to related kinases such as Src. The mechanistic basis for this became clear when the structure of the Abl kinase domain in complex with an imatinib analogue was solved (29). Contrary to expectations, imatinib was found to bind a unique inactive conformation of Abl while it was excluded from the active conformation, due to a sterical clash with the "activation loop" of the kinase, a flexible structure that controls access to the catalytic site (Fig. 3). In contrast to the active conformations of kinase

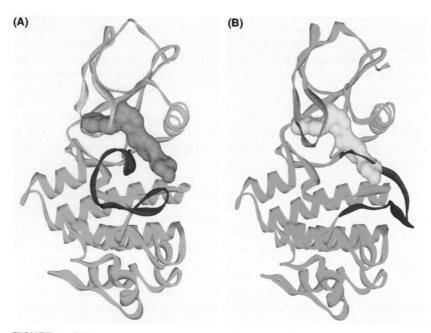

(A)   **(B)**

FIGURE 3 Ribbon representation of imatinib (IM) in complex with the kinase domain of Abl. (**A**) In the imatinib: Abl complex the activation loop (magenta) is in "closed" conformation, blocking the catalytic site for ATP and substrate binding. (**B**) Structure of Abl in an active conformation (green) with a surface representation of imatinib (yellow) superimposed. The activation loop is colored red and the glycine-rich or P-loop is colored orange. The N-methyl piperazine group of imatinib sits on the path of the activation loop in the active kinase, which is why imatinib cannot use this mode of binding for active Abl kinase (50). *Source*: Courtesy of Sandra W. Cowan-Jacob, Novartis Institutes of Biomedical Research, Basel, Switzerland.

domains that are quite similar across different tyrosine and even serine/threonine kinases, the inactive conformations are distinct, which explains imatinib's high degree of selectivity.

In preclinical studies imatinib demonstrated remarkable and specific activity against a variety of Bcr-Abl positive cell lines, including lines engineered to express Bcr-Abl and lines derived from blast crisis CML and Ph-positive ALL (30,31). Given that patient derived cell lines exhibit multiple genetic abnormalities, this was extremely encouraging and supported the view that Bcr-Abl kinase is an excellent therapeutic target. Importantly, selective suppression of colony formation by CML progenitor cells compared to normal progenitors was also demonstrated over a wide dose range (31). Finally, in vivo activity was demonstrated in a murine model using subcutaneous injection of Bcr-Abl positive cells (30).

CLINICAL TRIALS OF IMATINIB

The encouraging preclinical results led to the initiation of a phase I clinical trial in Spring of 1998. The initial study included patients with late chronic phase CML who had failed interferon-α, but was later extended to patients with accelerated phase and blast crisis. Significant clinical activity was demonstrated, including hematologic responses at doses of at least 140 mg daily and cytogenetic responses at doses of 300 mg or higher daily (32). Not surprisingly, responses were more consistent and durable in chronic phase compared to accelerated phase and blast crisis (33). The phase I study was rapidly followed by a series of phase II trials in patients with blast crisis, accelerated phase, and late chronic phase. These studies confirmed or surpassed the results of the phase I trial (34,35). Eventually, a phase III study compared imatinib with the drug therapy standard at the time, the combination of interferon-α and cytarabine. This trial demonstrated superiority of imatinib over the combination therapy in all major endpoints, including quality of life (36). Imatinib was approved by the regulatory authorities for the treatment of advanced CML in 2001 and newly diagnosed patients in 2003.

CONDITIONS FOR SUCCESSFUL MOLECULAR THERAPY

An important question arising from the remarkable success of imatinib therapy of CML is whether this success is the exception or the rule for targeted therapy of malignant disease. Time has told that the answer is neither. For example, overall results of clinical trials with specific inhibitors of the Flt3 kinase in AML were rather sobering (37). On the other hand, durable responses were seen with imatinib therapy in many patients with hypereosinophilic syndrome (38) and myeloproliferative diseases associated with activation of the platelet derived growth factor receptor (Pdgfr) kinase (39). Thus, what are the secrets of success and which factors are limiting?

1. *One lesion for one disease* CML is exceptional in the sense that the correlation between morphology and the presence of a particular genetic abnormality, *BCR-ABL*, is exceptionally tight. This has not only encouraged research into CML and facilitated the development of diagnostics, but also implies that clinical trials are easy to design, since they can draw on a rather homogeneous patient population. One would predict that kinase targeted therapy of polycythemia vera, where a V617F mutation of Jak2 is present in practically all

patients (40), will be equally successful. In contrast, AML is a heterogeneous disease, with subsets of patients carrying mutations of various tyrosine kinases or Ras. Thus, the design of clinical trials is naturally more complex, and sophisticated molecular testing and stratification is required to optimize the detection of clinical activity.

2. *Lesions of initiation versus lesions of progression.* One of the cardinal reasons for the disappointment about the results of clinical trials with Flt3 inhibitors in AML was the fact that expectations were far too optimistic, as they were based on the impressive results of imatinib in chronic phase CML (32). However, the more appropriate comparison would have been CML in blast crisis, where imatinib has only limited activity (33). Equally important, there is evidence that BCR-ABL initiates CML and is required for the maintenance of the leukemic cellular phenotype (15). In contrast, tyrosine kinase mutations may be a secondary event in AML. Evidence for this comes from the observation that FLT3 mutant clones have appeared or disappeared at the time of relapse in some patients, suggesting that their presence is limited to subclones and may be conducive to, but not essential, for the leukemic phenotype. Similarly, patients with AML1-ETO positive AML frequently have activating mutations of Kit. In patients with long-term remission after chemotherapy, clonogenic AML1-ETO positive cells but not mutant KIT positive cells have been shown to persist, suggesting that the KIT mutations were a secondary genetic event (41). In this situation, tyrosine kinase inhibitor-based therapy would not be expected to eradicate the disease but rather only induce regression to an earlier stage of disease evolution.

3. *Gain of function versus loss of function mutation.* One trivial but important consideration is that Bcr-Abl is a gain of function lesion and, hence, can be directly inhibited. This is therapeutically easier to tackle than restoring loss of function, for example, the inactivation of a tumor suppresser such as p53.

4. *Paucitargeted versus multitargeted inhibitors.* ABL knockout mice have a severe phenotype with very high neonatal lethality, and mice with a combined disruption of ABL and ARG (ABL related gene, also referred to as ABL-2) are embryonically lethal due to defects in neurulation (42). KIT is critical to hematopoietic development and PDGF to vascular development. Thus, one might expect that a drug that inhibits all these kinases will have significant side effects. Surprisingly and fortunately, this is not the case with imatinib. The precise reasons for the unexpectedly good tolerability of imatinib are unclear. One possibility is that the target kinases have lesser importance to the adult than to the developing organism. Alternatively, kinase activity is never inhibited to 100%, and residual activity may be sufficient to preserve vital functions in normal cells. In contrast to imatinib, tyrosine kinase inhibitors with broader activity spectrum, such as PKC412, have considerably more side effects than imatinib (43). The other side of the coin is the question whether some "off target" effects are actually desirable or not. In the case of imatinib, there is experimental evidence that targeting Kit along with Bcr-Abl may actually contribute to the effects of Abl inhibition in primary hematopoietic cells (44). If this were indeed the case, then imatinib would actually represent an extremely fortunate example of an inhibitor that targets two critical kinases,

simultaneously. To prove this point, it would be necessary to compare the clinical activity of imatinib with a "pure" Abl kinase inhibitor, a compound that does not currently exist. It is conceivable that in the future it may be possible to design drugs "a la carte" that are capable of simultaneously targeting several critical nodes in an oncogenic signal transduction network.

TARGETING *BCR-ABL* RATHER THAN ITS KINASE ACTIVITY

The fact that Bcr-Abl kinase activity is central to its transforming potency has served as the rationale for the development of imatinib for therapy of Bcr-Abl positive leukemias. There is some evidence that targeting the kinase activity may have limitations. Some biological effects of Bcr-Abl are not kinase dependent, including effects on migration and adhesion (19). While these effects obviously do not prevent imatinib from inducing responses, it remains possible that they contribute to the persistence of minimal residual disease. Thus, eliminating these cells would require agents that target the Bcr-Abl protein rather than its kinase activity. Compounds with this activity include geldanamycin derivatives, which inhibit heat-shock protein 90 (HSP90), a molecular chaperone required for Bcr-Abl stability (45), LAQ824, a histone deacetylase inhibitor (46), and arsenic trioxide (47). Another possibility is that, the survival of primitive CML stem cells is independent of Bcr-Abl, relying on physiological signals provided by the bone marrow microenvironment or cytokines. If this were the case, then neither inhibiting Bcr-Abl kinase activity nor eliminating the protein would be sufficient to eradicate residual leukemia (48). However, Bcr-Abl could still serve as a specific immunological target. In fact, Bcr-Abl junction peptides are processed by and expressed by CML mononuclear cells (49). This opens the possibility of developing vaccines to specifically target leukemia cells.

CONCLUSION

Bcr-Abl in CML, probably, represents the almost ideal molecular target. It defines the disease, has gain of function status, and is both necessary and sufficient for the initiation and maintenance of the disease phenotype. Few other malignant conditions have a similarly "simple" molecular make-up. One would predict that in these, imatinib's success will be repeatable, while most other malignant conditions will pose greater challenges to targeted therapy.

REFERENCES

1. SEER data 1996-2000. 2006. Type: Internet Communication
2. Heyssel R, Brill B, Woodbury L. Leukemia in Hiroshima bomb survivors. Blood 1960; 15:313.
3. Sawyers CL. Chronic myeloid leukemia. N Engl J Med 1999; 340:1330–1340.
4. Nowell P, Hungerford D. A minute chromosome in human chronic granulocytic leukemia. Science 1960; 132:1497.
5. Rowley JD. A new consistent chromosomal abnormality in chronic myelogenous leukaemia identified by quinacrine fluorescence and Giemsa staining. Nature 1973; 243:290–293.
6. Bartram CR, de Klein A, Hagemeijer A, et al. Translocation of c-abl oncogene correlates with the presence of a Philadelphia chromosome in chronic myelocytic leukaemia. Nature 1983; 306:277–280.

7. Groffen J, Stephenson JR, Heisterkamp N, et al. Philadelphia chromosomal breakpoints are clustered within a limited region, bcr, on chromosome 22. Cell 1984; 36:93–99.
8. Anafi M, Gazit A, Gilon C, Ben Neriah Y, Levitzki A. Selective interactions of transforming and normal abl proteins with ATP, tyrosine-copolymer substrates, and tyrphostins. J Biol Chem 1992; 267:4518–4523.
9. Vardiman JW, Pierre R, Thiele J, et al. Chronic myeloproliferative diseases. In: Jaffe ES, Harris NL, Stein H, Vardiman JW, eds. Tumors of Haematopoietic and Lymphoid Tissues. Lyon: IARCPress; 2001:15–59.
10. Melo JV. The diversity of BCR-ABL fusion proteins and their relationship to leukemia phenotype. Blood 1996; 88:2375–2384.
11. Van Etten RA. Cycling, stressed-out and nervous: cellular functions of c-Abl. Trends Cell Biol 1999; 9:179–186.
12. Tybulewicz VL, Crawford CE, Jackson PK, Bronson RT, Mulligan RC. Neonatal lethality and lymphopenia in mice with a homozygous disruption of the c-abl proto-oncogene. Cell 1991; 65:1153–1163.
13. Schwartzberg PL, Stall AM, Hardin JD, et al. Mice homozygous for the ablm1 mutation show poor viability and depletion of selected B and T cell populations. Cell 1991; 65:1165-1175.
14. Nagar B, Hantschel O, Young MA, et al. Structural basis for the autoinhibition of c-Abl tyrosine kinase. Cell 2003; 112:859–871.
15. Deininger MW, Goldman JM, Melo JV. The molecular biology of chronic myeloid leukemia. Blood 2000; 96:3343–3356.
16. Papadopoulos P, Ridge SA, Boucher CA, Stocking C, Wiedemann LM. The novel activation of ABL by fusion to an ets-related gene, TEL. Cancer Res 1995; 55:34–38.
17. Harnois T, Constantin B, Rioux A, et al. Differential interaction and activation of Rho family GTPases by p210bcr-abl and p190bcr-abl. Oncogene 2003; 22:6445–6454.
18. Castor A, Nilsson L, Astrand-Grundstrom I, et al. Distinct patterns of hematopoietic stem cell involvement in acute lymphoblastic leukemia. Nat Med 2005; 11:630–637.
19. Ramaraj P, Singh H, Niu N, et al. Effect of mutational inactivation of tyrosine kinase activity on BCR/ABL-induced abnormalities in cell growth and adhesion in human hematopoietic progenitors. Cancer Res 2004; 64:5322–5331.
20. Goss VL, Lee KA, Moritz A, et al. A common phosphotyrosine signature for the Bcr-Abl kinase. Blood 2006.
21. Gaston I, Johnson KJ, Oda T, et al. Coexistence of phosphotyrosine-dependent and -independent interactions between Cbl and Bcr-Abl. Exp Hematol 2004; 32:113–121.
22. Melo JV, Deininger MW. Biology of chronic myelogenous leukemia–signaling pathways of initiation and transformation. Hematol Oncol Clin North Am 2004; 18:545–viii.
23. Skorski T. BCR/ABL regulates response to DNA damage: the role in resistance to genotoxic treatment and in genomic instability. Oncogene 2002; 21:8591–8604.
24. Sexl V, Piekorz R, Moriggl R, et al. Stat5a/b contribute to interleukin 7-induced B-cell precursor expansion, but abl- and bcr/abl-induced transformation are independent of stat5. Blood 2000; 96:2277–2283.
25. Li S, Gillessen S, Tomasson MH, et al. Interleukin 3 and granulocyte-macrophage colony-stimulating factor are not required for induction of chronic myeloid leukemia-like myeloproliferative disease in mice by BCR/ABL. Blood 2001; 97:1442–1450.
26. Dinulescu DM, Wood LJ, Shen L, et al. c-CBL is not required for leukemia induction by Bcr-Abl in mice. Oncogene 2003; 22:8852–8860.
27. Sattler M, Mohi MG, Pride YB, et al. Critical role for Gab2 in transformation by BCR/ABL. Cancer Cell 2002; 1:479–492.
28. Hu Y, Liu Y, Pelletier S, et al. Requirement of Src kinases Lyn, Hck and Fgr for BCR-ABL1-induced B-lymphoblastic leukemia but not chronic myeloid leukemia. Nat Genet 2004; 36:453–461.
29. Schindler T, Bornmann W, Pellicena P, et al. Structural mechanism for STI-571 inhibition of abelson tyrosine kinase. Science 2000; 289:1938–1942.
30. Druker BJ, Tamura S, Buchdunger E, et al. Effects of a selective inhibitor of the Abl tyrosine kinase on the growth of Bcr-Abl positive cells. Nat Med 1996; 2:561–566.

31. Deininger M, Goldman JM, Lydon NB, Melo JV. The tyrosine kinase inhibitor CGP57148B selectively inhibits the growth of *BCR-ABL* positive cells. Blood 1997; 90:3691–3698.
32. Druker BJ, Talpaz M, Resta DJ, et al. Efficacy and safety of a specific inhibitor of the *BCR-ABL* tyrosine kinase in chronic myeloid leukemia. N Engl J Med 2001; 344:1031–1037.
33. Druker BJ, Sawyers CL, Kantarjian H, et al. Activity of a specific inhibitor of the *BCR-ABL* tyrosine kinase in the blast crisis of chronic myeloid leukemia and acute lymphoblastic leukemia with the Philadelphia chromosome. N Engl J Med 2001; 344:1038–1042.
34. Kantarjian H, Sawyers C, Hochhaus A, et al. Hematologic and cytogenetic responses to imatinib mesylate in chronic myelogenous leukemia. N Engl J Med 2002;346:645–652.
35. Talpaz M, Silver RT, Druker BJ, et al. Imatinib induces durable hematologic and cytogenetic responses in patients with accelerated phase chronic myeloid leukemia: results of a phase 2 study. Blood 2002; 99:1928–1937.
36. O'Brien SG, Deininger MW. Imatinib in patients with newly diagnosed chronic-phase chronic myeloid leukemia. Semin Hematol 2003; 40:26–30.
37. Wadleigh M, DeAngelo DJ, Griffin JD, Stone RM. After chronic myelogenous leukemia: tyrosine kinase inhibitors in other hematologic malignancies. Blood 2005; 105:22–30.
38. Gleich GJ, Leiferman KM, Pardanani A, Tefferi A, Butterfield JH. Treatment of hypereosinophilic syndrome with imatinib mesilate. Lancet 2002; 359:1577–1578.
39. Apperley JF, Gardembas M, Melo JV, et al. Response to imatinib mesylate in patients with chronic myeloproliferative diseases with rearrangements of the platelet-derived growth factor receptor beta. N Engl J Med 2002; 347:481–487.
40. James C, Ugo V, Le Couedic JP, et al. A unique clonal JAK2 mutation leading to constitutive signalling causes polycythaemia vera. Nature 2005; 434:1144–1148.
41. Wang YY, Zhou GB, Yin T, et al. AML1-ETO and C-KIT mutation/overexpression in t(8;21) leukemia: Implication in stepwise leukemogenesis and response to Gleevec. Proc Natl Acad Sci USA 2005; 102:1104–1109.
42. Koleske AJ, Gifford AM, Scott ML, et al. Essential roles for the Abl and Arg tyrosine kinases in neurulation. Neuron 1998; 21:1259–1272.
43. Stone RM, DeAngelo DJ, Klimek V, et al. Patients with acute myeloid leukemia and an activating mutation in FLT3 respond to a small-molecule FLT3 tyrosine kinase inhibitor, PKC412. Blood 2005; 105:54–60.
44. Wong S, McLaughlin J, Cheng D, et al. Sole *BCR-ABL* inhibition is insufficient to eliminate all myeloproliferative disorder cell populations. Proc Natl Acad Sci USA. 2004; 101:17456–17461.
45. An WG, Schulte TW, Neckers LM. The heat shock protein 90 antagonist geldanamycin alters chaperone association with p210bcr-abl and v-src proteins before their degradation by the proteasome. Cell Growth Differ 2000; 11:355–360.
46. Nimmanapalli R, Fuino L, Bali P, et al. Histone deacetylase inhibitor LAQ824 both lowers expression and promotes proteasomal degradation of Bcr-Abl and induces apoptosis of imatinib mesylate-sensitive or -refractory chronic myelogenous leukemia-blast crisis cells. Cancer Res 2003; 63:5126–5135.
47. La Rosee P, Johnson K, Corbin AS, et al. In vitro efficacy of combined treatment depends on the underlying mechanism of resistance in imatinib-resistant Bcr-Abl-positive cell lines. Blood 2004; 103:208–215.
48. Deininger MW, Holyoake TL. Can we afford to let sleeping dogs lie? Blood 2005; 105:1840–1841.
49. Clark RE, Dodi IA, Hill SC, et al. Direct evidence that leukemic cells present HLA-associated immuno genic peptides derived from the *BCR-ABL* b3a2 fusion protein. Blood 2001; 98:2887–2893.
50. Cowan-Jacob SW, Guez V, Fendrich G, et al. 2893. Imatinib (STI571) resistance in chronic myelogenous leukemia: molecular basis of the underlying mechanisms and potential strategies for treatment. Mini-Rev Med Chem 2004; 4:285–299.
51. Deininger and Melo Hematol Oncol Clin North Am 2004; 18(3):545–568.

2 Allogeneic Hematopoietic Stem Cell Transplantation for Chronic Myelogenous Leukemia

Mukta Arora
Department of Hematology, Oncology and Transplantation, University of Minnesota, Minneapolis, Minnesota, U.S.A.

Mary M. Horowitz
Department of Medicine, Center for International Blood and Marrow Transplant Research, Medical College of Wisconsin, Milwaukee, Wisconsin, U.S.A.

INTRODUCTION

Allogeneic hematopoietic stem cell transplantation (HCT) is currently the only treatment proven to cure chronic myelogenous leukemia (CML). Despite excellent response rates with few toxicities with imatinib, trials with this drug only began in 1998. The longest follow-up is now less than 10 years and there are relatively few patients who were followed more than five years on this therapy. Additionally, many continue to have molecular evidence of disease despite prolonged treatment (1–3). Consequently, duration of imatinib response remains somewhat uncertain. In contrast, there are now thousands of patients followed for more than 10 years (many for more than 15 and 20 years) after allogeneic HCT with documented persistent hematologic and molecular remissions (4–6). However, also in contrast to imatinib, HCT is associated with high rates of morbidity and mortality that limit its use in older patients and make it less appealing as front-line therapy even in young patients.

Not surprisingly, introduction of imatinib led to substantial changes in the use of HCT for CML. Prior to imatinib, CML treatment algorithms commonly called for early HCT in young patients with a human leukocyte antigen (HLA)-identical donor. Although the threshold for young varied by institution, most recommended HCT within one year of diagnosis in patients up to age 40 to 50 years with an HLA-identical sibling and in patients up to age 30 to 40 years with an HLA-identical unrelated donor. Patients considered at higher risk for transplant complications, either because of age or comorbidities, or patients without an HLA-identical donor often received a therapeutic trial of interferon. In the event of achieving major or complete cytogenetic response, HCT would frequently be deferred until there were signs of disease progression. If interferon failed to induce response, patients underwent allografting if a suitable alternative donor were available and there were no other contraindications. This changed after imatinib. In Europe, HCT for CML decreased by about 40% from 1999 to 2003 (6). Data from the Center for International Blood and Marrow Transplant Research (CIBMTR, formerly the International Bone Marrow Transplant Registry or IBMTR) indicate that the number of allografts for CML in the United States decreased by about two-thirds from 1999 to 2003. CML accounted for more than 25% of allogeneic HCTs done in the

United States in 1998—1999, but for fewer than 10% in 2003. Also, in 1999, fewer than 1% of HCT recipients had received imatinib at some time prior to transplantation compared to 77% in 2003. Despite these changes, most clinicians agree that HCT is a valuable treatment for some patients with CML, affording the possibility of cure in patients with high-risk disease or those failing imatinib therapy.

MECHANISM OF ACTION OF ALLOGENEIC TRANSPLANTATION

The general procedure for allogeneic HCT is to administer high (marrow ablative) doses of chemotherapy with or without radiation (pretransplant conditioning) to eradicate leukemia cells, followed by the infusion of healthy hematopoietic stem cells to restore hematopoiesis. The most common conditioning regimens employ high-dose cyclophosphamide combined with total body irradiation or with high-dose busulfan. Randomized comparisons of cyclophosphamide/total body irradiation and cyclophosphamide/busulfan in patients with chronic phase CML indicate similar efficacy and toxicity (4,7,8). That high-dose therapy helps to eradicate CML cells is supported by the finding that low blood levels of busulfan are associated with higher relapse rates and by the long-term remissions achieved with genetically identical twin transplantations (9,10). However, there are also considerable data supporting a critical role for allogeneic donor cells in controlling and/or curing CML (graft vs. leukemia or GVL effects) (10–20). These data include: (*i*) higher relapse rates after genetically identical twin compared to allogeneic transplantation (10,12); (*ii*) lower relapse rates in allotransplant recipients who develop graft-versus-host disease (GVHD, mediated by donor immune cells) (11,12,15); (*iii*) higher relapse rates when the donor graft is depleted of T-lymphocytes (12–16); and (*iv*) re-establishment of molecular remission after post-transplant relapse by stopping post-transplant immune suppression or infusing donor lymphocytes (17–20). The magnitude of these immune-mediated antileukemia effects is substantial. For example, allotransplant recipients with GVHD have a four-fold lower risk of leukemia relapse than those without GVHD. Recipients of identical twin transplants have a four-fold higher risk of CML relapse than allotransplant recipients. Available data suggest that GVL effects in CML are largely T-cell-mediated, but that only part of the effect requires development of clinically important GVHD.

OUTCOMES OF ALLOGENEIC TRANSPLANTATION
Transplantation from HLA-Matched Related Donors

The first successful HCT for CML was a bone marrow transplant from an identical twin donor, and was reported in 1979 (21). This was followed by transplants from HLA-identical sibling donors (22–24). In 1984, the IBMTR reported good outcomes in 117 patients undergoing HLA-identical sibling donor transplantation for CML (25). Three-year survival rates of 63%, 36%, and 12% were observed for patients transplanted in chronic, accelerated, and blast phases, respectively. In the 1990s, CML became the most frequent indication for allogeneic transplantation. Results improved over time. An analysis by the European Group for Blood and Marrow Transplantation (EBMT) divided patients into three time cohorts: 1980–1990, 1991–1999, and 2000–2003 (6). Two-year survival rates improved from 53% in the first time period to 61% in the most recent because of reduced transplant-related mortality. Relapse rates ranged from 14% to 22%. Among 3359 patients receiving HLA-identical sibling transplants for CML in 1998–2003 and reported to the CIBMTR, five-year probabilities of survival were (*i*) 73% for those transplanted in first chronic phase within one year of diagnosis; (*ii*) 60% for those transplanted in first chronic phase, but more than 12 months after diagnosis; (*iii*) 53% for those transplanted in accelerated phase; and 40% for those transplanted in blast phase (CIBMTR, unpublished data) (Fig. 1). Most post-transplant deaths occur early (within the first two years) and are due to transplant-related complications, such as infection, GVHD, and regimen-related toxicity (26). Reports with extended follow-up to 10 to 15 years indicate overall survival rates of 50% to 65% and disease-free survival rates of 45% to 50% for patients transplanted in chronic phase (27–30). In a meta-analysis of four randomized studies of 316 patients receiving HLA-identical sibling HCT in chronic phase, 10-year survival rates were 63% and 65% for patients receiving conditioning with cyclophosphamide/busulfan versus cyclophosphamide/total body irradiation, respectively, with relatively few events occurring after five years (4). A recent CIBMTR analysis of 2502 patients who were alive and in remission five years after HLA-identical sibling HCT for CML in chronic phase indicated a greater than 80% probability of surviving the subsequent 10 years, that is, to 15 years post-transplant (CIBMTR, unpublished data).

Several pretransplant patient and disease characteristics predict HCT outcomes. Factors independently associated with worse post-transplant survival are accelerated or blast phase disease, older age, and prolonged interval between diagnosis and HCT (24,31–34). A risk score for allogeneic HCT outcome was developed by the EBMT (35) and validated in a subsequent study by the CIBMTR (36). The latter study also validated the score in a separate analysis including only patients in early chronic phase. Factors significantly associated with survival and included in the score were patient age, interval between diagnosis and transplant, disease phase, donor-recipient sex-match, and donor type (Tables 1 and 2).

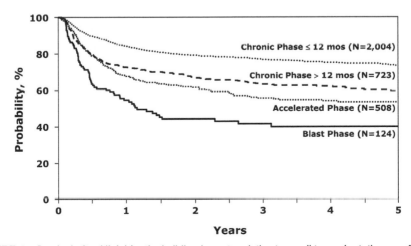

FIGURE 1 Survival after HLA-identical sibling hematopoietic stem cell transplantations performed in 1998–2003 and reported to the Center for International Blood and Marrow Transplant Research, by disease phase at time of transplantation.

TABLE 1 European Group for Blood and Marrow Transplantation Risk
Score for Patients with Chronic Myelogenous Leukemia

Prognostic factors	Risk score
Age	0 if <20 yrs
	1 if 20–40 yrs
	2 if >40 yrs
Interval from diagnosis to HSCT	0 if ≤1 yr
	1 if >1 yr
Disease phase	0 if chronic
	1 if accelerated
	2 if blast
Donor–recipient sex match	1 if female donor and male recipient
	0 if any other combination
Donor type	0 if HLA-identical sibling
	1 if any other

Abbreviations: HLA, human leukocyte antigen; HSCT, hematopoietic stem cell
transplant.

Transplantation from Unrelated Donors

HLA-identical sibling donors are available for fewer than 30% of otherwise eligible
transplant candidates. Unrelated donor transplantation can result in successful outcomes in patients with CML, although the transplant-related risks are higher than
with HLA-identical sibling donors. Overall, two- to three-year survival rates of 35%
to 45% are reported (16,37–44). In a series of 1423 transplants for CML facilitated by
the United States National Marrow Donor Program (NMDP), three-year leukemia-
free survival was 43% in 914 patients transplanted in first chronic phase (44). There
was a high incidence of severe acute GVHD (43%, grades II–IV; 33%, grades III–
IV). However, only 6% of patients relapsed, indicating a strong GVL effect.
Among 1724 patients receiving unrelated donor transplants for CML in 1998–
2003 and reported to the CIBMTR, five-year probabilities of survival were (*i*) 64%
for those transplanted in first chronic phase within one year of diagnosis; (*ii*) 59%
for those transplanted in first chronic phase, but more than 12 months after diagnosis; (*iii*) 43% for those transplanted in accelerated phase; and (*iv*) 29% for those
transplanted in blast phase (CIBMTR, unpublished data) (Fig. 2). The Fred Hutch-
inson Cancer Research Center reported outcomes in 196 patients with CML in
chronic phase, receiving transplants from unrelated donors (43). Overall survival

TABLE 2 Probability of Overall Survival at Five Years by
European Group for Blood and Marrow Transplantation
Risk Score

Risk score	Five-year overall survival (%)
0	72
1	70
2	62
3	48
4	40
5	18
6–7	22

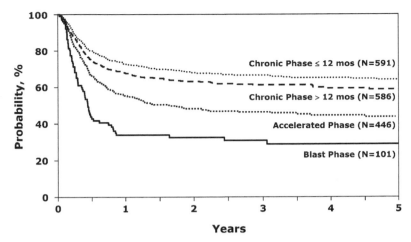

FIGURE 2 Survival after unrelated donor hematopoietic stem cell transplantations performed in 1998–2003 and reported to the Center for International Blood and Marrow Transplant Research, by disease phase at time of transplantation.

was 57% at five years. Thirty-five percent of patients developed severe (grades III–IV) GVHD. Only 10% of patients had leukemia relapse. Among patients aged 50 years or younger who received HCT within one year of diagnosis from an HLA-A, -B, and -DRB1 matched unrelated donor, five-year survival was 74%, which was similar to that observed after HLA-matched sibling transplants at the same center.

Post-transplant survival is correlated with identified risk factors. These include patient age, interval from diagnosis to transplantation, disease phase, CMV serostatus of the recipient, degree of donor–recipient HLA match, frequency of cytotoxic T-lymphocyte precursors in donor blood, and total nucleated cell dose of infused marrow (37–51). Results of unrelated donor transplantation in children with CML are similar to those in young adults. The EBMT Pediatric Disease Working Group reported outcomes in 44 children transplanted for CML between 1988 and 1995 (52). Long-term disease-free survival was 50%. Transplant-related mortality was high (38%), but few patients relapsed (7%).

In view of the high incidence of GVHD and associated transplant-related mortality, alternative approaches to unrelated donor transplantation have been explored. Depleting the graft of donor T-lymphocytes before infusion can decrease the incidence of GVHD, but at the cost of an increased risk of relapse, especially in patients with advanced disease (16,38,53–56). In a retrospective comparative analysis, outcomes in 46 patients with chronic phase CML receiving T-cell depleted transplants from an HLA-identical sibling donor were compared to outcome in 40 patients receiving non-T-cell depleted HLA-identical sibling transplants (54). Patients receiving T-cell depleted transplants had a lower incidence of acute and chronic GVHD and a somewhat lower incidence of transplant-related mortality than those receiving non-T-cell depleted transplants. However, the estimated three-year probability of relapse (cytogenetic or hematologic) was higher for patients receiving T-cell depleted versus non-T-cell depleted transplants (62% vs. 24%). Subsequent treatment with donor lymphocyte infusions resulted in remissions in 17 of the 20 patients relapsing after T-cell depleted transplants and the three-year probability of survival was similar in the two groups (72% vs. 68%). A large multicenter randomized trial of T-cell depleted versus non-T-cell depleted transplants from unrelated donors, sponsored by the United States National Heart Lung and Blood Institute, was performed in 1995–2000 (16). This trial enrolled 405 patients, of whom 182 were transplanted for CML in first chronic ($n = 160$), or accelerated, or second chronic ($n = 22$) phase. Patients receiving T-cell depleted transplants had lower risks of acute GVHD but higher risks of relapse. Among those with CML, the three-year probability of relapse was about 20% with a T-cell depleted but less than 10% with a non-T-cell depleted grafts. Probabilities of overall and leukemia-free survival were not significantly different with T-cell depleted and non-T-cell depleted grafts, both for the group as a whole and for the subgroup of patients with CML.

TREATMENT OF POST-TRANSPLANT RELAPSE

Although allogeneic HCT is successful in eradicating CML in most HCT recipients, post-transplant relapses do occur. The probability of relapse at five years is about 20% for patients receiving HLA-identical sibling transplants in first chronic phase (10–13,32,57). The risk is higher for patients transplanted in accelerated or blast phase varying from 20% in patients with both acute and chronic GVHD to 65% in patients without GVHD (11). Relapse rates are higher if the donor is an identical twin (where there is no allogeneic GVL effect) or if the graft is depleted of T-cells (which abrogates some or all of the GVL effect) (10–12,15,16).

Therapeutic options for patients who relapse following allogeneic HCT include infusions of donor lymphocytes (DLIs), second transplants with reduced intensity or myeloablative conditioning, and imatinib or IFN-a. Numerous studies support the use of DLI to exploit GVL effects to induce complete molecular remissions (17–20,58–62). Complete remissions can be established in up to 75% of patients, especially when DLIs are administered in early cytogenetic relapse (19,60). These remissions are durable with almost 90% persisting at two to three years after infusion. In an analysis reported by Collins et al. (20), complete responses were seen in 76% of patients receiving DLI for molecular or chronic phase hematologic relapse compared to 33% in patients with accelerated phase relapse and 17% in patients with blast phase relapse. Response rates are somewhat higher in patients who develop GVHD, but durable molecular responses occur in many patients without clinically evident GVHD. In the study by Collins et al. (20), 60% of patients developed GVHD and up to 20% of infusions were also complicated by marrow aplasia. Other data suggest that these complications can be ameliorated by infusion of lower numbers of cells, with dose increases in the case of nonresponse (58–61). However, the optimal dose and schedule for DLI are yet to be determined. The effect of the initial cell dose (mononuclear cells $\times 10^8/kg$ received in the first infusion) on outcome was retrospectively analyzed in 298 of 344 patients treated with DLI at 51 centers (61). Patients were classified into three groups according to the initial cell dose: <0.20, 0.21–2.0, and >2.0 (mononuclear cells $\times 10^8/kg$). Additional infusions were given to 62%, 20%, and 5% of patients in the three groups, respectively. Response rates were similar in the three groups (78%, 73%, and 70%, respectively). However, a lower initial cell dose was associated with less GVHD (26%, 53%, and 62%), less myelosuppression (10%, 23%, and 24%), less DLI-related mortality (5%, 20%, and 22%), and higher three-year leukemia-free survival (66%, 57%, and 45%).

This suggests that starting with a low dose reduces the toxicity of DLI, although dose escalation may be necessary to achieve a response.

Second hematopoietic stem cell transplantation with full or reduced intensity conditioning is sometimes used for post-transplant relapse, but is associated with high rates of transplant-related mortality, especially if the interval between the first and second transplant is less than one year. This approach is generally reserved for young patients who relapse with accelerated or blast phase CML more than a year after a first transplant.

Imatinib is also reported to be an effective treatment for post-transplant CML relapse in small case series (62–66). Olavarria et al. reported outcomes in 128 patients receiving imatinib after relapsing after allogeneic HCT. Fifty-one patients were in chronic phase, 31 in accelerated phase, and 46 in blast crisis (66). Fifty patients had failed treatment with DLI prior to imatinib. The overall hematological response rate was 84%. The complete cytogenetic response rate was 58% for patients in chronic phase, 48% for those in accelerated phase, and 22% for those in blast crisis. Twenty-five (26%) patients had complete molecular responses. With median follow-up of nine months, the estimated probabilities of two-year survival were 100%, 86%, and 12% for patients treated in chronic phase, accelerated phase, and blast crisis, respectively. These results are encouraging, but longer follow-up is necessary. Additionally, treatment with imatinib in these patients is not without side effects, particularly cytopenias. Future studies are needed to help clarify the role of imatinib with and without DLI for CML relapse following allogeneic HCT.

LATE EFFECTS IN SURVIVORS

As noted earlier, patients who survive the first five years after HCT are likely to survive long-term with mortality rates eventually approaching that of the general population (5). However, some survivors experience late complications of HCT. Baker et al. (67) studied the long-term risks and benefits of HCT for CML. Two hundred forty-eight recipient of HCT for CML who had survived at least two years post-HCT were compared to 317 normal siblings. Subjects completed a 238-item survey on medical late effects. When compared with sibling controls, survivors had higher risks of ocular, oral health, endocrine, gastrointestinal, musculoskeletal, neurosensory, and neuromotor impairments. Multivariate analysis of the allograft recipients identified chronic GVHD as a major risk factor for hypothyroidism, osteoporosis, cardiopulmonary, neurosensory, and neuromotor impairments. These data show the need for continued monitoring and medical intervention in these patients. The CIBMTR and EBMT recently published guidelines for long-term follow-up of transplant recipients (68).

NEW APPROACHES TO ALLOGENEIC TRANSPLANTATION
Reduced Intensity Conditioning
The most important recent strategy to decrease the early morbidity and mortality of HCT is the use of reduced intensity conditioning (69–73). This approach uses immunosuppressive, but not myeloablative, doses of drugs and radiation to allow donor cell engraftment and relies upon the GVL effects of allografting to eradicate CML. The reduced intensity of conditioning drugs is intended to decrease the incidence of regimen-related toxicity and, by decreasing the extent of tissue

injury and release of inflammatory cytokines, reduce the severity of GVHD. The EBMT has reported outcomes in 187 patients receiving reduced intensity conditioning followed by allogeneic HCT between 1994 and 2002 (72). The median age was 50 years. Sixty-one percent received a transplant from an HLA-identical sibling donor, 25% from an unrelated, and the remainder from HLA-mismatched related donors. Transplant-related mortality was only 6% at 100 days but rose to 23% by two years post-transplant, still lower than expected with standard myeloablative conditioning regimens. Grades II–IV acute GVHD occurred in 32%, and chronic GVHD in 43% of patients. Among patients transplanted in first or second chronic phase, overall and leukemia-free survivals at three years were 69% and 57%, respectively. Two-year survivals of patients transplanted in accelerated or blast phase were only 24% and 8%, respectively. Progressive CML was the major cause of death. Among 368 patients receiving HLA-identical sibling transplants after reduced intensity conditioning in 2000–2005 and reported to the CIBMTR, the three-year probabilities of relapse, survival, and leukemia-free survival were 39%, 72%, and 52%, respectively. Follow-up of these patients is relatively short and, consequently, duration of remissions uncertain at present. However, early results are sufficiently encouraging to consider this approach in patients unable to tolerate standard conditioning because of age or comorbidities.

Umbilical Cord Blood Transplantation

One important obstacle to allografting is identifying a suitable donor for 70% of patients without an HLA-identical sibling. Currently about 25% of these patients receive a transplant from an adult unrelated volunteer identified through the NMDP or another of the national and international donor registries. Successful transplants are also reported using umbilical cord blood (74–78). The major advantage of cord blood in this setting is a lesser requirement for stringent HLA-matching, increasing the likelihood of finding a unit that is suitable in terms of HLA. The major drawback of this approach is the limited number of cells in each cord blood unit, such that not all adults will find a unit with a suitable cell dose which leads to slow rates of hematopoietic recovery relative to bone marrow or peripheral blood transplants. A recent analysis compared outcomes following 150 unrelated cord blood and 450 unrelated adult donor bone marrow transplants in patients with leukemia (74). Twenty-five percent of the cord blood recipients and 40% of the bone marrow recipients had CML. All of the cord blood transplants were one ($n = 34$) or two ($n = 116$) HLA-antigen mismatched; in 367 patients the bone marrow transplants were HLA-matched and 83 were one-antigen mismatched. Hematopoietic recovery was slower with cord blood (27 days) than with HLA-matched (18 days) or mismatched (20 days) marrow transplants. Acute but not chronic GVHD was less likely with cord blood transplantation. Rates of transplant-related mortality, treatment failure, and overall mortality were lowest among patients who received HLA-matched marrow transplants. Patients who received one antigen mismatched marrow transplants and those who received one or two antigen mismatched cord blood transplants had similar rates of transplant-related mortality, treatment failure, and overall mortality. Results were similar in patients with acute leukemia and those with CML. These data indicate that a one or two antigen mismatched cord blood transplant may be an acceptable alternative for patients who need HCT but do not have an HLA-identical adult donor, extending the possibility of HCT to many more persons in need. Studies are in progress to develop approaches to facilitate engraftment with limited cord blood cell doses, including use of multiple units and cell expansion techniques.

INDICATIONS FOR HEMATOPOIETIC STEM CELL TRANSPLANTATION

Since HCT is the only therapy with documented molecular remissions lasting more than 20 years, the possibility of this intervention, with its attendant risks and benefits, should be discussed with young patients presenting with CML. Although imatinib is the first-line therapy of choice, consultation with a transplant physician is advised to evaluate the potential role of HCT (including performing a preliminary related and unrelated donor search), to formulate a strategy for HCT in the event of imatinib failure and agree upon a strategy for monitoring the patient's progress. Early HCT is indicated for patients whose initial presentation is in blast phase and should be considered for those with a suboptimal response to imatinib. HCT should also be considered for patients whose CML progresses after an initial response. Careful monitoring for early signs of progression is indicated since outcomes are significantly better if HCT is performed prior to transformation to accelerated or blast phase. Definitions of suboptimal response and failure with imatinib, guidelines for monitoring patients on imatinib, and indications for initiating alternative therapy, including HCT, were recently developed and published by a consensus panel sponsored by the European LeukemiaNet (79).

REFERENCES

1. Kantarjian H, Sawyers C, Hochhaus A, et al. Hematologic and cytogenetic responses to imatinib mesylate in chronic myelogenous leukemia. N Engl J Med 2002; 346:645–652.
2. O'Brien SG, Guilhot F, Larson RA, et al. Imatinib compared with interferon and low-dose cytarabine for newly diagnosed chronic-phase chronic myeloid leukemia. N Engl J Med 2003; 348:994–1004.
3. Hahn EA, Glendenning GA, Sorensen MV, et al. Quality of life in patients with newly diagnosed chronic phase chronic myeloid leukemia on imatinib versus interferon alfa plus low-dose cytarabine: results from the IRIS Study. J Clin Oncol 2003; 21:2138–2146.
4. Socie G, Clift RA, Blaise D, et al. Busulfan plus cyclophosphamide compared with total-body irradiation plus cyclophosphamide before marrow transplantation for myeloid leukemia: long-term follow-up of 4 randomized studies. Blood 2001; 98:3569–3574.
5. Socié G, Veum-Stone J, Wingard JR, et al. Long-term survival and late deaths after allogeneic bone marrow transplantation. N Engl J Med 1999; 341:14–21.
6. Gratwohl A, Brand R, Apperley J, et al. Allogeneic hematopoietic stem cell transplantation for chronic myeloid leukemia in Europe 2006: transplant activity, long-term data and current results. An analysis by the Chronic Leukemia Working Party of the European Group for Blood and Marrow Transplantation (EBMT). Haematologica 2006; 91:513–521.
7. Clift RA, Buckner CD, Appelbaum FR, et al. Allogeneic marrow transplantation in patients with chronic myeloid leukemia in the chronic phase: a randomized trial of two irradiation regimens. Blood 1991; 77:1660–1665.
8. Clift RA, Radich J, Appelbaum FR, et al. Long-term follow-up of a randomized study comparing cyclophosphamide and total body irradiation with busulfan and cyclophosphamide for patients receiving allogenic marrow transplants during chronic phase of chronic myeloid leukemia. Blood 1999; 94:3960–3962.
9. Slattery JT, Clift RA, Buckner CD, et al. Marrow transplantation for chronic myeloid leukemia: the influence of plasma busulfan levels on the outcome of transplantation. Blood 1997; 89:3055–3060.
10. Gale RP, Horowitz MM, Ash RC, et al. Identical-twin bone marrow transplants for leukemia. Ann Intern Med 1994; 120:646–652.

11. Sullivan KM, Weiden PL, Storb R, et al. Influence of acute and chronic graft-versus-host disease on relapse and survival after bone marrow transplantation from HLA-identical siblings as treatment of acute and chronic leukemia. Blood 1989; 73: 1720–1728.

12. Horowitz MM, Gale RP, Sondel PM, et al. Graft-versus-leukemia reactions after bone marrow transplantation. Blood 1990; 75:555–562.

13. Marmont AM, Horowitz MM, Gale RP, et al. T-cell depletion of HLA-identical transplants in leukemia. Blood 1991; 78:2120–2130.

14. Marks DI, Hughes TP, Szydlo R, et al. HLA-identical sibling donor bone marrow transplantation for chronic myeloid leukaemia in first chronic phase: influence of GVHD prophylaxis on outcome. Br J Haematol 1992; 81:383–390.

15. Enright H, Davies SM, DeFor T, et al. Relapse after non-T-cell-depleted allogeneic bone marrow transplantation for chronic myelogenous leukemia: early transplantation, use of an unrelated donor, and chronic graft-versus-host disease are protective. Blood 1996; 88:714–720.

16. Wagner JE, Thompson JS, Carter SL, Kernan NA. Effect of graft-versus-host disease prophylaxis on 3-year diseases-free survival in recipients of unrelated donor bone marrow (T-cell Depletion Trial): a multi-centre, randomised phase II-III trial. Lancet 2005; 366:733–741.

17. van Rhee F, Lin F, Cullis JO, et al. Relapse of chronic myeloid leukemia after allogeneic bone marrow transplant: the case for giving donor leukocyte transfusions before the onset of hematologic relapse. Blood 1994; 83:3377–3383.

18. Kolb HJ, Schattenberg A, Goldman JM, et al. Graft-versus-leukemia effect of donor lymphocyte transfusions in marrow grafted patients. Blood 1995; 86:2041–2050.

19. Porter DL, Roth MS, McGarigle C, Ferrara JL, Antin JH. Induction of graft-versus-host disease as immunotherapy for relapsed chronic myeloid leukemia. N Engl J Med 1994; 330:100–106.

20. Collins RH Jr, Shpilberg O, Drobyski WR, et al. Donor leukocyte infusions in 140 patients with relapsed malignancy after allogeneic bone marrow transplantation. J Clin Oncol 1997; 15:433–444.

21. Fefer A, Cheever MA, Thomas ED, et al. Disappearance of Ph1-positive cells in four patients with chronic granulocytic leukemia after chemotherapy, irradiation and marrow transplantation from an identical twin. N Engl J Med 1979; 300:333–337.

22. Clift RA, Buckner CD, Thomas ED, et al. Treatment of chronic granulocytic leukaemia in chronic phase by allogeneic marrow transplantation. Lancet 1982; 2:621–623.

23. Goldman JM, Baughan AS, McCarthy DM, et al. Marrow transplantation for patients in the chronic phase of chronic granulocytic leukaemia. Lancet 1982; 2:623–625.

24. Speck B, Gratwohl A, Nissen C, et al. Allogeneic marrow transplantation for chronic granulocytic leukemia. Blut 1982; 45:237–242.

25. Speck B, Bortin MM, Champlin R, et al. Allogeneic bone-marrow transplantation for chronic myelogenous leukaemia. Lancet 1984; 1:665–668.

26. Passweg JR, Rowlings PA, Horowitz MM. Related donor bone marrow transplantation for chronic myelogenous leukemia. Hematol Oncol Clin North Am 1998; 12:81–92.

27. Monitoring treatment and survival in chronic myeloid leukemia. Italian Cooperative Study Group on Chronic Myeloid Leukemia and Italian Group for Bone Marrow Transplantation. J Clin Oncol 1999; 17:1858–1868.

28. Gratwohl A, Brand R, Apperley J, et al. Graft-versus-host disease and outcome in HLA-identical sibling transplantations for chronic myeloid leukemia. Blood 2002; 100:3877–3886.

29. Simonsson B, Oberg G, Bjoreman M, et al. Intensive treatment and stem cell transplantation in chronic myelogenous leukemia: long-term follow-up. Acta Haematol 2005; 113:155–162.

30. Robin M, Guardiola P, Devergie A, et al. A 10-year median follow-up study after allogeneic stem cell transplantation for chronic myeloid leukemia in chronic phase from HLA-identical sibling donors. Leukemia 2005; 19:1613–1620.

31. Biggs JC, Szer J, Crilley P, et al. Treatment of chronic myeloid leukemia with allogeneic bone marrow transplantation after preparation with BuCy2. Blood 1992; 80:1352–1357.

32. Goldman JM, Szydlo R, Horowitz MM, et al. Choice of pretransplant treatment and timing of transplants for chronic myelogenous leukemia in chronic phase. Blood 1993; 82:2235–2238.
33. Clift RA, Buckner CD, Thomas ED, et al. Marrow transplantation for patients in accelerated phase of chronic myeloid leukemia. Blood 1994; 84:4368–4373.
34. Enright H, Daniels K, Arthur DC, et al. Related donor marrow transplant for chronic myeloid leukemia: patient characteristics predictive of outcome. Bone Marrow Transplant 1996; 17:537–542.
35. Gratwohl A, Hermans J, Goldman JM, et al. Risk assessment for patients with chronic myeloid leukaemia before allogeneic blood or marrow transplantation. Chronic Leukemia Working Party of the European Group for Blood and Marrow Transplantation. Lancet 1998; 352:1087–1092.
36. Passweg JR, Walker I, Sobocinski KA, Klein JP, Horowitz MM, Giralt SA. Validation and extension of the EBMT Risk Score for patients with chronic myeloid leukaemia (CML) receiving allogeneic haematopoietic stem cell transplants. Br J Haematol 2004; 125:613–620.
37. McGlave P, Bartsch G, Anasetti C, et al. Unrelated donor marrow transplantation therapy for chronic myelogenous leukemia: initial experience of the National Marrow Donor Program. Blood 1993; 81:543–550.
38. Drobyski WR, Ash RC, Casper JT, et al. Effect of T-cell depletion as graft-versus-host disease prophylaxis on engraftment, relapse, and disease-free survival in unrelated marrow transplantation for chronic myelogenous leukemia. Blood 1994; 83:1980–1987.
39. Davies SM, Ramsay NK, Haake RJ, et al. Comparison of engraftment in recipients of matched sibling of unrelated donor marrow allografts. Bone Marrow Transplant 1994; 13:51–57.
40. Davies SM, Shu XO, Blazar BR, et al. Unrelated donor bone marrow transplantation: influence of HLA A and B incompatibility on outcome. Blood 1995; 86:1636–1642.
41. Spencer A, Szydlo RM, Brookes PA, et al. Bone marrow transplantation for chronic myeloid leukemia with volunteer unrelated donors using ex vivo or in vivo T-cell depletion: major prognostic impact of HLA class I identity between donor and recipient. Blood 1995; 86:3590–3597.
42. Devergie A, Apperley JF, Labopin M, et al. European results of matched unrelated donor bone marrow transplantation for chronic myeloid leukemia. Impact of HLA class II matching. Chronic Leukemia Working Party of the European Group for Blood and Marrow Transplantation. Bone Marrow Transplant 1997; 20:11–19.
43. Hansen JA, Gooley TA, Martin PJ, et al. Bone marrow transplants from unrelated donors for patients with chronic myeloid leukemia. N Engl J Med 1998; 338:962–968.
44. McGlave PB, Shu XO, Wen W, et al. Unrelated donor marrow transplantation for chronic myelogenous leukemia: 9 years' experience of the national marrow donor program. Blood 2000; 95:2219–2225.
45. Craddock C, Szydlo RM, Dazzi F, et al. Cytomegalovirus seropositivity adversely influences outcome after T-depleted unrelated donor transplant in patients with chronic myeloid leukaemia: the case for tailored graft-versus-host disease prophylaxis. Br J Haematol 2001; 112:228–236.
46. Spencer A, Brookes PA, Kaminski E, et al. Cytotoxic T lymphocyte precursor frequency analyses in bone marrow transplantation with volunteer unrelated donors. Value in donor selection. Transplantation 1995; 59:1302–1308.
47. O'Shea J, Madrigal A, Davey N, et al. Measurement of cytotoxic T lymphocyte precursor frequencies reveals cryptic HLA class I mismatches in the context of unrelated donor bone marrow transplantation. Transplantation 1997; 64:1353–1356.
48. Szydlo R, Goldman JM, Klein JP, et al. Results of allogeneic bone marrow transplants for leukemia using donors other than HLA-identical siblings. J Clin Oncol 1997; 15:1767–1777.
49. Petersdorf EW, Longton GM, Anasetti C, et al. The significance of HLA-DRB1 matching on clinical outcome after HLA-A, B, DR identical unrelated donor marrow transplantation. Blood 1995; 86:1606–1613.

50. Petersdorf EW, Gooley TA, Anasetti C, et al. Optimizing outcome after unrelated marrow transplantation by comprehensive matching of HLA class I and II alleles in the donor and recipient. Blood 1998; 92:3515–3520.

51. Pocock C, Szydlo R, Davis J, et al. Stem cell transplantation for chronic myeloid leukaemia: the role of infused marrow cell dose. Hematol J 2001; 2:265–272.

52. Dini G, Rondelli R, Miano M, et al. Unrelated-donor bone marrow transplantation for Philadelphia chromosome-positive chronic myelogenous leukemia in children: experience of eight European Countries. The EBMT Paediatric Diseases Working Party. Bone Marrow Transplant 1996; 18(suppl 2):80–85.

53. Hessner MJ, Endean DJ, Casper JT, et al. Use of unrelated marrow grafts compensates for reduced graft-versus-leukemia reactivity after T-cell-depleted allogeneic marrow transplantation for chronic myelogenous leukemia. Blood 1995; 86:3987–3996.

54. Sehn LH, Alyea EP, Weller E, et al. Comparative outcomes of T-cell-depleted and non-T-cell-depleted allogeneic bone marrow transplantation for chronic myelogenous leukemia: impact of donor lymphocyte infusion. J Clin Oncol 1999; 17:561–568.

55. Drobyski WR, Hessner MJ, Klein JP, et al. T-cell depletion plus salvage immunotherapy with donor leukocyte infusions as a strategy to treat chronic-phase chronic myelogenous leukemia patients undergoing HLA-identical sibling marrow transplantation. Blood 1999; 94:434–441.

56. Zander AR, Kroger N, Schleuning M, et al. ATG as part of the conditioning regimen reduces transplant-related mortality (TRM) and improves overall survival after unrelated stem cell transplantation in patients with chronic myelogenous leukemia (CML). Bone Marrow Transplant 2003; 32:355–361.

57. Apperley JF, Mauro FR, Goldman JM, et al. Bone marrow transplantation for chronic myeloid leukaemia in first chronic phase: importance of a graft-versus-leukaemia effect. Br J Haematol 1988; 69:239–245.

58. Mackinnon S, Papadopoulos EB, Carabasi MH, et al. Adoptive immunotherapy evaluating escalating doses of donor leukocytes for relapse of chronic myeloid leukemia after bone marrow transplantation: separation of graft-versus-leukemia responses from graft-versus-host disease. Blood 1995; 86:1261–1268.

59. Giralt S, Hester J, Huh Y, et al. CD8-depleted donor lymphocyte infusion as treatment for relapsed chronic myelogenous leukemia after allogeneic bone marrow transplantation. Blood 1995; 86:4337–4343.

60. Chiorean EG, DeFor TE, Weisdorf DJ, et al. Donor chimerism does not predict response to donor lymphocyte infusion for relapsed chronic myelogenous leukemia after allogeneic hematopoietic cell transplantation. Biol Blood Marrow Transplant 2004; 10:171–177.

61. Guglielmi C, Arcese W, Dazzi F, et al. Donor lymphocyte infusion for relapsed chronic myelogenous leukemia: prognostic relevance of the initial cell dose. Blood 2002; 100:397–405.

62. Olavarria E, Craddock C, Dazzi F, et al. Imatinib mesylate (STI571) in the treatment of relapse of chronic myeloid leukemia after allogeneic stem cell transplantation. Blood 2002; 99:3861–3862.

63. Savani BN, Montero A, Kurlander R, Childs R, Hensel N, Barrett AJ. Imatinib synergizes with donor lymphocyte infusions to achieve rapid molecular remission of CML relapsing after allogeneic stem cell transplantation. Bone Marrow Transplant 2005; 36:1009–1015.

64. Kantarjian HM, O'Brien S, Cortes JE, et al. Imatinib mesylate therapy for relapse after allogeneic stem cell transplantation for chronic myelogenous leukemia. Blood 2002; 100:1590–1595.

65. DeAngelo DJ, Hochberg EP, Alyea EP, et al. Extended follow-up of patients treated with imatinib mesylate (gleevec) for chronic myelogenous leukemia relapse after allogeneic transplantation: durable cytogenetic remission and conversion to complete donor chimerism without graft-versus-host disease. Clin Cancer Res 2004; 10:5065–5071.

66. Olavarria E, Ottmann OG, Deininger M, et al. Response to imatinib in patients who relapse after allogeneic stem cell transplantation for chronic myeloid leukemia. Leukemia 2003; 17:1707–1712.

67. Baker KS, Gurney JG, Ness KK, et al. Late effects in survivors of chronic myeloid leukemia treated with hematopoietic cell transplantation: results from the Bone Marrow Transplant Survivor Study. Blood 2004; 104:1898–1906.
68. Rizzo JD, Wingard JR, Tichelli A, et al. G. Recommended screening and preventive practices for long-term survivors after hematopoietic cell transplantation: joint recommendations of the European Bone Marrow Transplant Group, Center for International Blood and Marrow Transplant Research, and the American Society of Blood and Marrow Transplantation. Biol Blood Marrow Transplant 2006; 12:138–151.
69. Bornhauser M, Kiehl M, Siegert W, et al. Dose-reduced conditioning for allografting in 44 patients with chronic myeloid leukaemia: a retrospective analysis. Br J Haematol 2001; 115:119–124.
70. Or R, Shapira MY, Resnick I, et al. Nonmyeloablative allogeneic stem cell transplantation for the treatment of chronic myeloid leukemia in first chronic phase. Blood 2003; 101:441–445.
71. Weisser M, Schleuning M, Ledderose G, et al. Reduced-intensity conditioning using TBI (8 Gy), fludarabine, cyclophosphamide and ATG in elderly CML patients provides excellent results especially when performed in the early course of the disease. Bone Marrow Transplant 2004; 34:1083–1088.
72. Baron F, Maris MB, Storer BE, et al. HLA-matched unrelated donor hematopoietic cell transplantation after nonmyeloablative conditioning for patients with chronic myeloid leukemia. Biol Blood Marrow Transplant 2005; 11:272–279.
73. Crawley C, Szydlo R, Lalancette M, et al. Outcomes of reduced-intensity transplantation for chronic myeloid leukemia: an analysis of prognostic factors from the Chronic Leukemia Working Party of the EBMT. Blood 2005; 106:2969–2976.
74. Laughlin MJ, Eapen M, Rubinstein P, et al. Outcomes after transplantation of cord blood or bone marrow from unrelated donors in adults with leukemia. N Engl J Med 2004; 351:2265–2275.
75. Barker JN, Weisdorf DJ, DeFor TE, et al. Transplantation of 2 partially HLA-matched umbilical cord blood units to enhance engraftment in adults with hematologic malignancy. Blood 2005; 105:1343–1347.
76. Wagner JE, Barker JN, DeFor TE, et al. Transplantation of unrelated donor umbilical cord blood in 102 patients with malignant and nonmalignant diseases: influence of CD34 cell dose and HLA disparity on treatment-related mortality and survival. Blood 2002; 100:1611–1618.
77. Laughlin MJ, Barker J, Bambach B, et al. Hematopoietic engraftment and survival in adult recipients of umbilical-cord blood from unrelated donors. N Engl J Med 2001; 344:1815–1822.
78. Gluckman E, Rocha V, Boyer-Chammard A, et al. Outcome of cord-blood transplantation from related and unrelated donors. Eurocord Transplant Group and the European Blood and Marrow Transplantation Group. N Engl J Med 1997; 337:373–381.
79. Baccarani M, Saglio G, Goldman J, et al. Evolving concepts in the management of chronic myeloid leukemia. Recommendations from an expert panel on behalf of the European LeukemiaNet. Blood May 2006; 108:1809–1820.

3 Where Are We Today with Imatinib Therapy?

John M. Goldman
Hematology Branch, National Institutes of Health,
Bethesda, Maryland, U.S.A.

INTRODUCTION

There has been considerable progress in recent years in the management of malignant disease in general, but in no other area has the progress been quite as remarkable as in the management of chronic myeloid leukemia (CML). We have seen the disease move from a status where chemotherapy changed the natural history little if at all to a time when selected patients could be treated and often "cured" by allogeneic stem cell transplantation (allo-SCT). Most recently we have witnessed the introduction of molecularly targeted therapy in the form of imatinib mesylate (IM), which offers the prospect of very substantial prolongation of life for the majority of patients, so much so that it has displaced transplant as primary therapy for newly diagnosed patients.

The pharmaceutical company Ciba-Geigy (now Novartis) initiated a program in the early 1990s to identify small molecules for clinical use that might inhibit relevant tyrosine kinases (1). One possible target, regarded as promising by some but by no means by all investigators at the time, was the *BCR-ABL* gene in CML. After some years during which the lead compound, a 2-phenylaminopyrimidine, was subjected to extensive chemical modification, an agent CGP57148B was developed that was intended for clinical use (2,3). Preclinical studies showed that it selectively inhibited the proliferation of Ph-positive CML cell lines and colony formation by Ph-positive myeloid progenitor cells while leaving proliferation of control cells unaffected (4–6). It was also active against tumors formed by Bcr-Abl expressing cells in a murine model system (4), although complete eradication of such tumors depended on continuous exposure to the agent over longer periods of time (7). These and other studies laid the foundation for the initial clinical trials, which started in the United States in June 1998.

RESULTS IN PREVIOUSLY TREATED PATIENTS

The initial phase I study of IM recruited patients with CML who were refractory or resistant to interferon-α (IFN) or intolerant of this agent. The study patients began at an oral dose of 25 mg daily that was escalated in increments to a maximum of 1000 mg daily. The drug half-life was 13 to 16 hours. The drug appeared to be well tolerated and a maximally tolerated dose was not defined. Of the 54 patients who had failed interferon-α and received IM at doses of 300 mg daily or higher, 53 (98%) achieved complete hematologic responses and the majority of responses lasted more than one year (8). In 38 patients with myeloid blast crisis, 21 (55%) responded at imatinib doses of 300 mg/day or greater, but the duration of response for these patients was usually limited (9).

TABLE 1 Inclusion Criteria for Patients in Phase II Studies

Chronic phase
  <15% blasts, <20% basophils in blood and BM, <30% blasts plus
  promyelocytes in blood and BM, platelets >100 × 10⁹/L
Accelerated phase
  + at least 15% and less than 30 blasts in PB or BM
  + at least 30% blasts plus promyelocytes in PB or BM
  + at least 20% basophils in PB
  + platelets <100 × 10⁹/L unrelated to therapy
Blastic phase
  + at least 30% blasts in PB or BM (confirmed by flow cytometry)
  + extramedullary evidence of CML

Abbreviations: BM, bone marrow; CML, chronic myeloid leukemia; PB, peripheral blood.

TABLE 2 Response Rates in Phase II Studies

	Chronic phase (n = 454)	Accelerated phase (n = 181)	Myeloid blast crisis (n = 229)
CHR	430 (95%)	96 (53%)	20 (9%)
MCyR	272 (60%)	43 (24%)	37 (15%)
CCyR	188 (41%)	30 (17%)	17 (7%)
Disease progression	47 (11%)	78 (43%)	183 (80%)

Abbreviations: CCyR, complete cytogenetic responses; CHR, complete hematologic response; MCyR, major cytogenetic responses.
Source: Adapted from Refs. 8,11,12.

    Thereafter a series of phase II studies was initiated for CML patients in chronic phase (CP) who satisfied criteria for interferon-α resistance or intolerance and for patients in advanced phases. In the CP study, 552 patients were treated with IM at 400 mg/day in six different countries over a period of six to nine months (10). The incidence of complete cytogenetic responses (CCyR) was 41%. In the accelerated phase study, 181 patients with confirmed CML were treated with IM at either 400 or 600 mg daily and 17% achieved a CCyR (11). For the 260 patients with myeloid blast crisis the overall response rate was 52%; 18% of patients had partial or complete hematologic responses and 7% had CCyRs (12). The median survival from starting IM treatment was six to nine months. These last results were appreciably better than those achievable with standard chemotherapy (13,14). The criteria for defining the various phases on CML were fairly standard (Table 1), and the response rates are summarized in Table 2.

PHASE III STUDY FOR NEWLY DIAGNOSED CHRONIC PHASE PATIENTS

From June 2000 until January 2001 a phase III study recruited a total of 1106 newly diagnosed patients with CML in CP for a clinical trial referred to as the International Randomized Study of Interferon and STI571 or IRIS (15). Equal numbers of patients received either IM at a dose of 400 mg daily or the combination of interferon-α(IFN) plus cytarabine. The two cohorts were essentially similar with regard to age, starting leukocyte counts, Sokal prognostic scores, and interval from diagnosis. At a median follow-up of 19 months, the estimated rate of major cytogenetic response for the patients who received IM was very much higher than the rate for the patients who received interferon-α and cytarabine (87.1 % vs. 34.7%, $P < 0.001$); similarly the estimated rates of CCyR were better in the IM-treated patients than in control patients (76.2% vs. 14.5%, $P < 0.001$). Freedom from progression to advanced phase disease was 97.7% for the imatinib patients and 91.5% for the control patients ($P < 0.001$). When progression was more broadly defined by any of the following—loss of response to treatment, increasing leukocyte count, onset of advanced phase, or death—the "broad" progression-free survival for IM-treated patients was again very significantly better than that of patients in the control arm. It was also of interest to note that sub-classification of patients into one of three prognostic categories according to criteria established by Sokal et al. (16) separated patients' progression-free survivals in both treatment arms, but progression-free survival for patients in all three Sokal categories was better for IM-treated patients than progression-free survival for patients in the best Sokal category treated with the control combination ($P < 0.01$).

The most recent analysis of results in the IRIS study was performed at a median follow-up of 60 months from initiation of treatment, at which point 382 (69%) of the 553 patients originally allocated to the IFN/cytarabine arm had crossed over to the IM arm in contrast to crossover in the reverse direction by only 14 (2.5%) patients. Some patients crossed over from the IFN/cytarabine arm on account of intolerance or failure to achieve complete hematologic response or major cytogenetic response by the predetermined target dates, but a major reason for discontinuing treatment with IFN/cytarabine was withdrawal of consent when IM was approved by the Food and Drug Administration (FDA) and other national regulatory agencies and so became available for general use. This high level of discontinuation of treatment in the control arm meant that clinical results could not be analyzed at five years as a conventional prospective study, but analysis of results of primary treatment with IM and comparisons of IM-treated patients with the control arm on an "intention-to-treat" basis were still highly informative. At a median follow-up of five years the clinical results appeared to have improved very substantially in comparison with results reported at 19 months (17). The estimated incidence of CCyR was 87% (Fig. 1); only 7% of patents had progressed to advanced phase. The estimated overall survival for all patients who had received IM as first-line therapy was 89% (Fig. 2), which contrasted with an overall survival of 82% for patients in the control arm, many of whom had actually switched to IM soon after starting the IFN/cytarabine combination to which they had originally been allocated. Landmark analyses performed at 12 and 18 months showed very clearly that the degree to which the total quantity of leukemia in a patient's body had been reduced, as assessed by marrow cytogenetic status and *BCR-ABL* transcript numbers in the blood at the two time points, was highly predictive of the probability of subsequent survival without progression to advanced phase disease (Fig. 3). Thus patients who had a more than 3-log reduction in *BCR-ABL* transcript numbers at 18 months compared with a standardized baseline value (see Chapter 4) had 99% survival without progression at five years, whereas patients who had failed to achieve CCyR had a corresponding value of 83%. ($P < 0.001$). Of even greater interest was the observation that in the IM cohort the annual rate of progression seemed to be diminishing from year one to year five (Table 3), and similarly for patients who achieved CCyR the annual rate of progression to advanced phase seemed to be diminishing from year one to year four (17).

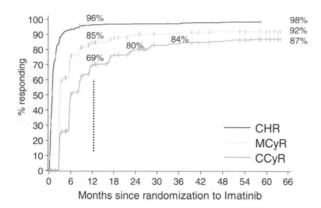

FIGURE 1 Probability of achieving complete hematological response, major cytogenetic response and complete cytogenetic response for 553 patients randomized to receive imatinib mesylate at 400 mg/day as initial treatment for chronic myeloid leukemia in chronic phase in the International Randomized Study of Interferon and STI571 study. The dashed vertical line shows values at one year from start of therapy. *Abbreviations*: CCyR, complete cytogenetic response; CHR, complete hematologic response; MCyR, major cytogenetic response.

SURVIVAL COMPARED WITH HISTORICAL CONTROL PATIENTS

In the absence of results of a formal prospective assessment of survival for patients in CP who received IM compared with that of contemporary patients who received optimal alternative therapy, a comparison of survival for patients who received IM with survival for historical control patients who received IFN or IFN plus other agents is warranted. The Houston group compared results of treating 261 patients

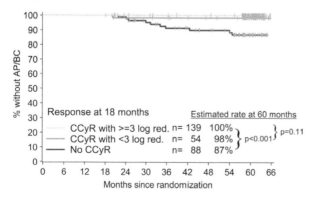

FIGURE 2 Landmark analysis of projected survival without progression to advanced phase disease for patients treated with imatinib mesylate 400 mg/day as initial therapy in the International Randomized Study of Interferon and STI571 classified at 18 months from start of therapy according to whether they had achieved: (*i*) complete cytogenetic responses (CCyR) with more than 3 log reduction in *BCR-ABL* transcripts, (*ii*) CCyR with less than 3 log reduction in *BCR-ABL* transcripts, or (*iii*) no CCyR. It is notable that patients in category (*i*) had an estimated 100% freedom from disease progression at five years from start of therapy. *Abbreviations*: CML, chronic myeloid leukemia; CI, confidence interval.

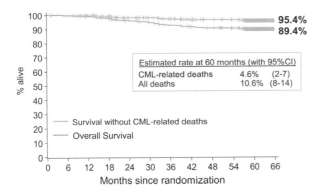

FIGURE 3 Estimated survival at five years for patients with chronic myeloid leukemia (CML) in chronic phase who started treatment with imatinib at 400 mg/day in the International Randomized Study of Interferon and STI571 study. Deaths were classified as (*i*) attributable to CML or (*ii*) due to any cause, including CML. *Abbreviations*: AP, accelerated phase; BC, blastic phase; CCyR, complete cytogenetic response.

with CML in CP who received IM after failing IFN with results in 204 patients with similar disease status who had received optimal therapy, most of which included interferon alone or in combination with other agents, in the preimatinib era (18). The CCyR rates were 62% and 19%, respectively, in the IM versus historical control arms ($P < 0.001$); survival at two years from beginning treatment with IM was 93% compared with 71% for patients in the control arm ($P < 0.001$). The Hammersmith group compared survival for 143 patients who received IM after prior treatment with interferon-α with survival for 246 patients treated before IM was available, primarily with IFN. They reported a significant survival advantage for patients who received IM, but noted that this applied only to patients who achieved some degree of cytogenetic response after six months on the new drug (19).

The Houston group also had the opportunity to compare survival for 187 patients in early CP who received IM with that of a historical control group of 650 patients treated predominantly with IFN-α. At median follow-up of 19 months, survival with IM therapy was significantly better than survival for patients in the control group ($P < 0.01$). Survival for all IM-treated patients was also significantly better than survival for the Sokal good risk subset in the control arm (20). In a recent update of this original study the group compared results of treating 279 newly diagnosed patients with IM with the original 650 patients treated with interferon. The CCyR rates were 87% with IM and 28% with interferon-α ($P < 0.0001$). The estimated three-year survival rates were 96% with IM and 81% with IFN-α ($P < 0.01$) (21). A collaborative study group in France compared survival of patients whose primary treatment was IM in the IRIS study with survival for 325 patients who received the combination of IFN-α plus cytarabine in the French multicenter CML91 trial, which recruited patients between 1991 and 1996 (22). With a follow-up of 42 months for both patient groups, the estimated incidence of CCyR, of survival without progression to advanced phase by three years and of overall survival at three years were all significantly better in the IM group than in the historical control population (81% vs. 32%, $P < 0.0001$; 90% vs. 82%, $P < 0.04$; and 92% vs. 84%, $P < 0.0001$, respectively).

TABLE 3 Incidence of progression (*i*) Broadly Defined, and (*ii*) to advanced phase for 553 Patients with Chronic Myeloid Leukemia in Chronic Phase Allocated to Receive Imatinib as Primary Treatment

Year	Progression[a] (%)	AP/BP[b] (%)
1st	3.4	1.5
2nd	7.5	2.8
3rd	4.8	1.6
4th	1.5	0.9
5th	0.9	0.6

[a]Progression includes all deaths and all patients who lost their response to imatinib, including progression to advanced phase.
[b]AP/BP includes patients who progressed to advanced phase (accelerated phase and/or blastic phase).
Abbreviations: AP, accelerated phase; BP, blastic phase.

PREDICTING RESPONSE TO IMATINIB

Although the molecular characteristics of *BCR-ABL*−positive CML seem at present to be remarkably similar in different patients, it is widely accepted that the disease is in fact highly heterogeneous. Thus Sokal et al. (16) in the 1980s were able to categorize CML patients treated with busulfan into three prognostic groups based on criteria defined at diagnosis, and Hasford et al. (23) in the 1990s carried out a similar exercise with patients treated predominantly with IFN-α. The observed differences might theoretically have been due principally to the fact that the disease was diagnosed in different patients at different points of its natural history (24,25), but it is intuitively more likely that the differences reflect differences intrinsic to the kinetics of the disease in a given patient (26). This view gains some support from the observation that 15% to 20% of patients whose leukemia cells have a deletion of genetic sequences in the vicinity of the *ABL-BCR* gene on the derivative chromosome 9q+ had a survival inferior to those lacking this deletion in the preimatinib era (27,28), although the adverse effect of the 9q+ deletion is not apparent in the IM-treated patients (29,30).

Micro-array studies of CD34+ cells collected at diagnosis from two subgroups of patients distinguished on the basis of whether their subsequent disease course was relatively short or much longer than average showed very different gene expression patterns (31), further supporting the notion of genetic heterogeneity. Despite the fact that there is a general agreement that the pattern of gene expression may differ substantially according to the phase of disease (32–35), it has proved more difficult to identify genes differentially expressed in patients who respond and patients who do not respond well to imatinib (36), but one recent study has shown that patients who relapse after initial response to IM have a gene expression profile more closely resembling advanced phase than CP disease (35). It is most probable that this technology will soon prove useful for defining prognosis.

In the laboratory, the enhanced kinase activity of the $p210^{Bcr-Abl}$ is most reproducibly reflected by its capacity to phosphorylate the substrate CrkL, although the pathogenetic significance of this observation remains obscure. The Adelaide group has recently reported that the IM IC_{50} as measured by in vitro inhibition of CrkL phosphorylation correlates with clinical response. In other words patients with a low IC_{50}s for IM had superior clinical responses to those with relatively high IC_{50}s (37). Although these preliminary studies were based on relatively small numbers of patients and used mononuclear cells separated from the blood of newly diagnosed patients, the approach seems very promising. They need to be confirmed with larger numbers of patients and appropriate cell fractions, for example, CD34+ cells or CD34+ CD38− cells. Moreover, this approach now needs to be extended to define IC_{50}s for the newer TK inhibitors.

Somewhat simpler than using Crkl as the target for measuring phosphorylation by Bcr-Abl is measurement of total phosphotyrosine levels in a target cell population. Inhibition of total phosphotyrosine by IM is a reliable indicator of the effect of IM in cell lines (38). The use of an antiphosphotyrosine antibody in conjunction with cytofluorimetry to measure phosphotyrosine levels in CD34+ cells exposed to IM showed that IM responders had significantly higher levels of inhibition than nonresponding patients (39). These preliminary observations were based on relatively small numbers of patients and should now be expanded to confirm their applicability to larger number of patients treated with IM 400 or 800 mg daily.

Interest has focused on the possibility that responses to IM could differ in different patients as a result of intrinsic difference in the manner which leukemia stem cells handle the drug. The ATP-binding cassette reporters, notably MDR1, ABC1 and ABCG2, are involved act as ATP-dependent efflux pumps and could all theoretically contribute to reducing intracellular concentration of IM. There is evidence that MDR1 over expression could be a basis for CML cell resistance to IM (38,40), but a recent study of ABCG2 showed that though CML CD34+ cells over-express functional ABCG2, IM is not a substrate but rather inhibits this transporter molecule (41). Conversely, the organic cationic transporter-1 (OCT1) provides an active mechanism for influx of a number of drugs and seems to be involved in entry into cells of IM. The Liverpool group reported that influx of IM into CML cell lines depended on intracellular levels of OCT1 (42), and the Oregon group showed highly significant positive correlation between cellular OCT1 levels and response to IM in individual patients (43). Interestingly, response to nilotinib seems not to depend on OCT1 for intracellular transport (44). These studies focus attention on the possibility that influx and efflux of IM could explain differential responses in patients who receive comparable doses of the drug.

DEFINITIONS OF RESPONSE AND RESPONSE FAILURE

The sequence of events in CML patients responding to treatment with IM parallels closely the pattern in patients responding to other agents, but with the notable difference that the response to IM at 400 mg/day seems extremely rapid (and at higher dosage even more rapid). Thus the leukocyte counts start to fall rapidly and may reach normal values within 10 to 15 days, the percentage of Ph-positive marrow metaphases also falls such that the patients may be 100% Ph-negative within three months (or earlier) and the number of *BCR-ABL* transcripts continues to fall and reaches its nadir months or even years later. Thus, theoretically, one should be able to define a response based on hematologic, cytogenetic, or molecular criteria achieved at different time-points after starting imatinib. These criteria would also be sensitive to drug dosage, and the time-points would have to be adjusted for patients who start treatment with doses in excess of 400 mg/day.

In principle, resistance to IM may be primary or secondary and its definition must take account of (*i*) the quantity of leukemia in a patient's body as measured indirectly by blood counts, bone marrow cytogenetics, or the number of residual *BCR-ABL* transcripts in the blood or marrow, (*ii*) the dose of IM that the patient is taking, and (*iii*) the duration of treatment. Thus, in general, for the newly diagnosed patient with CML in CP who starts treatment at a "standard" dose of 400 mg/day, the patient should be able to satisfy specified criteria of response at various time points. Failure to achieve such levels would be attributable to "primary resistance" and would allow the patient to be classified as "failure" (Table 4). This would indicate the need to consider a change in therapeutic strategy, which could for example in some cases involve simply increasing the dose of imatinib. A patient who initially responds to IM but then loses the response should be classified as secondary failure. Thus, for example, a patient who after having

TABLE 4 Operational Definition of Failure and Suboptimal Response for Previously Untreated, ECP, Chronic Myeloid Leukemia Patients Who Are Treated with Imatinib Mesylate 400 mg/Day Proposed by Baccarani et al. on Behalf of the European LeukemiaNet

Time	Failure	Suboptimal response	Warnings
Diagnosis	NA	NA	High risk Del9q + ACA in Ph-positive cells
3 months	No HR (stable disease or disease progression)	Less than CHR	
6 months	Less than complete HR (CHR) No CyR (Ph-positive more than 95%)	Less than PCyR (Ph-positive more than 35%)	
12 months	Less than PCyR (Ph-positive more than 35%)	Less than CCyR	Less than MMR
18 months	Less than CCyR	Less than MMR	
Any time	Loss of CHR[a]	ACA in Ph-positive cells[d]	Any rise in transcript level
	Loss of CCyR[b]	Loss of MMR[d]	Other chromosome abnormalities in Ph-negative cells
	Mutation[c]	Mutation[e]	

Note: *Failure* implies that the patient should be moved to other treatments whenever available. *Suboptimal response* implies that the patient may still have a substantial benefit from continuing imatinib mesylate treatment, but that the long-term outcome is not likely to be optimal, so that the patient becomes eligible for other treatments. *Warnings* imply that the patient should be monitored very carefully and may become eligible for other treatments. The same definitions can be used to define the response after imatinib mesylate dose escalation.
[a]To be confirmed on two occasions unless associated with progression to accelerated phase (AP)/blast crisis (BC).
[b]To be confirmed on two occasions, unless associated with complete hematologic response loss or progression to AP/BC.
[c]High level of insensitivity to imatinib mesylate.
[d]To be confirmed on two occasions, unless associated with complete hematologic response or complete cytogenetic response loss.
[e]Low level of insensitivity to imatinib mesylate.
Abbreviations: ACA, additional chromosome abnormalities; CCyR, complete cytogenetic response; CyR, cytogenetic response; CHR, complete hematologic response; ECP, early chronic phase; HR, hematologic response; MMR, major molecular response; NA, not applicable; PCyR, partial cytogenetic response.
Source: Adapted from Ref. 46.

achieved hematologic control subsequently has a rising leukocyte or platelet count would satisfy criteria for secondary resistance. Similarly, a rising proportion of Ph-positive metaphases in the bone marrow or a rising number of BCR-ABL transcripts in a patient who had previously responded at cytogenetic or molecular levels would be classified as secondarily resistant. In all cases the clinician must be assured that a patient who satisfies criteria for failure is actually taking the drug at the specified dosage, since noncompliance, which is not uncommon, should not be mistaken for true resistance.

In 2003, the Hammersmith group attempted somewhat arbitrarily to define a series of features that would allow the clinician to say that an individual patient had failed to respond to treatment with imatinib at standard dosage (400 mg/day) or having responded had begun to lose his/her response (45). More recently, Baccarani, on behalf of colleagues in the European LeukemiaNet, has proposed that patients undergoing treatment with IM should be sub-classified according to whether they are high-risk before treatment onset and according to how they respond or lose their response after beginning treatment (Table 4) (46). According to these recommendations patients classified as "failure" should receive alternative therapy, patients classified as "sub-optimal response" should be considered for alternative therapy, and other patients may show features classifiable as "warnings." Patients in the last category do not necessary need a change of therapy, but should be monitored more closely than average.

In practice, the definition of failure may prove to be difficult in individual patients. For example, patients who proceed only very slowly to CCyR and subsequently to major molecular response may miss established milestones, but may still have a good overall prognosis (47). Moreover, it is likely that whereas some patients will continue to manifest reduction in transcript numbers during the first four years of therapy with imatinib, in other cases transcript numbers monitored sequentially may reach a plateau consistent with cytogenetic negativity or major molecular response (48). Should such patients be classified as resistant and offered alternative therapy? At this stage probably not.

MANAGING THE RESPONDER

Various lines of evidence suggest that even in patients who appear to have responded well to therapy and have achieved low or undetectable levels of BCR-ABL transcripts, some residual leukemia cells survive (49). First, investigators in Glasgow defined a "quiescent" leukemia stem cell on the basis of high Ph-positivity in association with retention of high levels of the fluorochrome CFSE (carboxyfluorescein succinimidyl ester), and showed that it appears to be unaffected by incubation with imatinib in vitro (50,51). Secondly, investigators in Los Angeles showed that some colonies cultured from CFU-GM collected from the marrow of patients in cytogenetic remission expressed a BCR-ABL gene (52). Thirdly, the observation that occasional patients in cytogenetic remission with undetectable BCR-ABL transcripts may progress abruptly to blastic phase disease (53,54) also suggests that at least in these patients CML had not been eradicated. Fourthly, further support for the notion that residual disease persists in "successfully" treated patients comes from the observation that even in patients who have had BCR-ABL transcripts undetectable for months or years, stopping imatinib is usually, though not always, associated with gradual recurrence of detectable transcripts (55–57).

There is currently no agreement about how best to manage the patient who responds well to IM. It was believed at one time that autografting might be useful both for the patient who relapsed on treatment with IM and for the patient who remained in CCyR. For this reason Ph-negative progenitor cells were collected from the peripheral blood of patients (58), but such cells have in practice been used only very rarely and the approach has largely fallen into disfavor. One could argue a case both for increasing the dose of IM and for reducing the dose of or for adding other drugs, such as interferon-α or cytarabine. Such patients could still benefit from some immunotherapeutic approach, such as vaccination with Bcr-Abl, Wt1 or Pr3 oligopeptides (59–62), or intact irradiated K562 cells engineered to produce GM-CSF (63). In practice, the simplest approach is probably to continue IM at standard dosage.

MANAGING THE NONRESPONDER

There are a number of possible therapeutic strategies for managing the patient who starts treatment with IM at 400 mg/day for CML in CP but then manifests primary or secondary resistance, but currently there is no general consensus. For example, a patient who in the pre-imatinib era would have been considered a candidate for allogeneic stem cell transplant could be offered a transplant after the patient has failed imatinib. Conversely, the patient could be offered treatment with one of the second generation tyrosine kinase inhibitors, namely dasatinib or nilotinib. Patients whose relapse is associated with a substantial sub-clone bearing a T315I mutation will prove resistant to these agents, but may respond to one of the third generation agents that target components of the Bcr-Abl protein other than the ATP-binding domain. Treatment with other agents known to be effective in CML, such as interferon-α, hydroxyurea, or busulfan, is a third option, but clinical results are not likely to be any better than was reported with use of these agents at the end of the last century. Resistant patients who still have low levels of residual disease could be considered for one of the new immunotherapeutic strategies mentioned earlier.

IMATINIB IN PATIENTS WHO RELAPSE AFTER ALLOGENEIC STEM CELL TRANSPLANTATION

The incidence of relapse after allo-SCT depends on a number of factors, including the phase of disease at the time of transplant, the nature of the conditioning regimen, the degree of histocompatibility between donor and recipient, and the techniques used to prevent or minimize GvHD. It is probable also that features intrinsic in the patient's disease are also relevant, although there is no definite association between Sokal score and probability of relapse. Until recently the standard approach to managing a patient with CML who relapsed after allo-SCT was to infuse lymphocytes (donor lymphocyte infusions, DLI) collected from the original transplant donor. However, recent experience shows that such relapses respond very well to IM, but the disease frequently recurs when the imatinib is discontinued (64,65). This may mean that DLI has a more durable effect than IM and the decision whether to use IM, DLI or a combination of both in a given patient may be difficult.

IMATINIB IN COMBINATION WITH OTHER AGENTS

Four or five years ago the longer term benefits of IM could not be predicted with any precision, so a number of clinical trials were designed to test the benefits of using other antileukemia agents in conjunction with IM. Most of these phase I/II clinical trials were based on in vitro studies suggesting potential synergism between IM and existing as well as investigational agents (66). These studies include amongst others combining IM, usually at full dosage with interferon-α (67), cytarabine (68), 5-aza-2'-deoxycytidine (decitabine) (69), farnesyl transferase inhibitors (70,71), homoharringtonine (72), and arsenic trioxide (73).

TOXICITY

IM administered to patents with CML is not without side effects, which may be classified as hematologic or nonhematologic. Both categories are for the most part manageable and only infrequently necessitate abandoning the use of the drug.

Patients who previously received treatment with IFN-α and sustain grade 3 or 4 neutropenia or thrombocytopenia on IM generally have a lower incidence of major or complete cytogenetic remission and shorter progression free survival than those without hematologic toxicity (74–76). The outlook for newly diagnosed patients who sustain major degrees of hematologic toxicity is not necessarily inferior to that of those who tolerate the drug well. Neutropenia can be managed by administration G-CSF as often as is required to maintain a neutrophil count above 1.0×10^9/L. Paradoxically thrombocytopenia may on occasion also respond to G-CSF. Persisting severe cytopenias will necessitate altering IM administration. Because of the possibility that administering the IM at daily doses less than 300 mg may induce resistance, it is currently conventional either to reduce the dose from 400 to 300 mg/day (but no lower) or temporarily to interrupt administration entirely and to resume treatment when the neutrophil count has risen again. Anemia attributable to IM usually responds to administration of erythropoietin and should not therefore be an indication for modifying drug dosage. It is notable that patients who received IM as treatment for gastrointestinal stromal tumors do not experience any significant hematologic toxicity, an observation that implies that the cytopenias seen in CML must be due to some inadequacy of residual normal hematopoiesis.

The list of side effects experienced by patients taking IM at 400 mg/day is extensive and includes edema, nausea, muscle cramps, bone pains, rashes, fatigue, headache, hemorrhage, and vomiting (77). Only a few of the symptoms have occurred with any frequency at grades 3 or 4; fatigue and depression have been the most common. The fluid retention often takes the form of infraorbital edema, but it may on rare occasion be more generalized. It usually responds to treatment with diuretics. In some cases where side effects have been attributed to IM and the drug was interrupted, it can safely be resumed under short-term cover of corticosteroids. In other cases the patients should be judged as "intolerant" and must therefore be treated by others means. Abnormal liver chemistry with raised hepatic enzymes occurs with some frequency and should be monitored closely, since the hepatic disturbance may progress and rare deaths attributable to hepatic failure in association with IM have been reported (78). Very rarely death due to cerebral edema has been attributed to IM (79).

CHOICE OF INITIAL TREATMENT FOR THE NEWLY DIAGNOSED PATIENT WITH CHRONIC MYELOID LEUKEMIA

Until the year 2000, the general policy for managing a newly diagnosed patient with CML in CP was to offer initial treatment by allo-SCT if the patient was young enough and had a suitable HLA-matched related or unrelated donor. The introduction of reduced intensity conditioning allo-SCT (also called nonmyeloablative transplants) enlarged the number of patients to whom allo-SCT could be offered. IM was first used in 1998 and it was some while before the durability of the responses was fully recognized (80). In the last few years however hematologists worldwide have generally adopted the view that all newly diagnosed adults with CML in CP should receive initial therapy with IM or an IM-containing combination. The optimal dose if IM is used as a single agent is not established and the possibility that patients may benefit from administration of IM conjunction with other agents is under study in various clinical trials. For the patient not in a clinical study, it is reasonable to initiate treatment with IM 400 mg/daily or possibly 600 mg/daily.

The situation for children is more complicated. Some pediatric hematologists believe that the capacity of allo-SCT to cure patients with CML means that a successful allo-SCT would be preferable to life-long treatment with IM; others feel that the longer term results of treatment with IM or second generation tyrosine kinase inhibitors may be so good that to subject even a child to the risks inherent in an allo-SCT is no longer justifiable.

The majority of patients who present today with CML in advanced phase will have received imatinib during their preceding CP and further administration of IM has no logical basis. However, the valuable short term results of treating IM-naïve patients with CML in advanced phase with higher dose of IM (11,12) suggest that this is a reasonable initial approach to the management of such patients. The analogy with results of treating patients presenting with Ph-positive acute lymphoblastic leukemia with the combination of IM and conventional cytotoxic drugs (81,82) suggests that this may be a valuable approach also for patients who present de novo with CML in accelerated or blastic phases.

CONCLUSIONS

The introduction of IM has changed very fundamentally the approaches to initial management of CML, but has also redirected the search for new agents that may be active in treating and eventually eradicating other forms of malignant disease. The story that has evolved over the last ten or more years has taught us some valuable lessons. First, where the "initiating genetic lesion" in a given neoplasm is reasonably well defined, molecular targeting can be impressively effective. Indeed, the incidence of "acquired" resistance to IM seems to diminish with time. Secondly, CML after its initial stage appears to accrue additional genetic changes, both in the *BCR-ABL* gene and in other genes in the Ph-positive clone, some of which may be innocuous and others of which may underlie increased resistance to a given agent. This must mean that treatment should be initiated at the earliest opportunity, a conclusion that may well generalize to other neoplastic conditions. Thirdly, drugs can be designed to deal effectively with some but currently not with all these additional mutations. It is likely however that combinations of inhibitory molecules can be designed that will broaden the efficacy of specific treatment regimens, and some such strategies are now being tested in the clinic. Fourthly, leukemia stem cells may be able to escape eradication by a drug that targets the protein they express, either because their quiescent status makes them "immune" to the effects of the drug or because such stem cells have intrinsic mechanisms that inactivate or prevent influx of the drug. Although it has been generally accepted that this failure to eradicate residual stem cells will mean that the disease must inexorably recur at some stage in the future, this might not be the case if the progeny of these residual stem cells retained sensitivity to imatinib. It now seems very possible that CML has been changed from a disease that was inevitably fatal to one that may be controlled long-term by relatively simple and nontoxic therapy. Once again, CML leads the way to revision of thinking about other neoplastic diseases and about the pharmacological strategies that may culminate in cure.

REFERENCES

1. Zimmermann J, Buchdunger E, Mett H, et al. Phenylaminopyrimidine (PAP)-derivatives: a new class of potent and highly selective PDGF receptor autophosphorylation inhibitors. Biorg Chem Med Lett 1996; 6:1221–1226.
2. Druker BJ, Lydon NB. Lessons learned from the development of an Abl tyrosine kinase inhibitor for chronic myelogenous leukemia. J Clin Invest 2000; 105:3–7.
3. Deininger M, Buchdunger E, Druker BJ. The development of imatinib as a therapeutic agent for chronic myeloid leukemia. Blood 2005; 105:2640–2653.
4. Druker BJ, Tamura S, Buchdunger E, et al. Effects of a selective inhibitor of the Abl tyrosine kinase on the growth of Bcr-Abl positive cells. Nature Medicine 1996; 2:561–566.
5. Deininger M, Goldman JM, Lydon NB, Melo JV. The tyrosine kinase inhibitor CGP57148B selectively inhibits the growth of BCR-ABL positive cells. Blood 1997; 90:3691–3698.
6. Gambacorti-Passerini C, le Coutre P, Mologni L, et al. Inhibition of the ABL kinase activity blocks the proliferation of BCR/ABL+ leukemic cells and induces apoptosis. Blood Cells Mol Dis 1997; 23:380–394.
7. Le Coutre P, Molgni L, Cleris L, et al. In vivo eradication of human BCR/ABL-positive leukemia cells with an ABL kinase inhibitor. J Natl Cancer Inst 1999; 91:163 168.
8. Druker BJ, Talpaz M, Resta D, et al. Efficacy and safety of a specific inhibitor of the Bcr-Abl tyrosine kinase in chronic myeloid leukemia. N Engl J Med 2001; 344:1031–1037.
9. Druker BJ, Sawyers CL, Kantarjian H, et al. Activity of a specific inhibitor of the Bcr-Abl tyrosine kinase in the blast crisis of chronic myeloid leukemia and acute lymphoblastic leukemia with the Philadelphia chromosome. N Engl J Med 2001; 344:1038–1042.
10. Kantarjian H, Sawyers C, Hochhaus A, et al. Hematologic and cytogenetic responses to imatinib mesylate in chronic myelogenous leukemia. N Engl J Med 2002; 346:645–652.
11. Talpaz M, Silver RT, Druker BJ, et al. Imatinib induces durable hematologic and cytogenetic responses in patients with accelerated phase chronic myeloid leukemia: results of a phase 2 study. Blood 2002; 99:1928–1937.
12. Sawyers CL, Hochhaus A, Feldman E, et al. Imatinib induces hematologic and cytogenetic responses in patients with chronic myelogenous leukemia in myeloid blast crisis: results of a phase II study. Blood 2002; 99:3530–3539.
13. Sacchi S, Kantarjian H, O'Brien S, et al. Chronic myelogenous leukemia in nonlymphoid blastic phase: analysis of the results of first salvage therapy with three different treatment approaches in 162 patients. Cancer 1999; 86:2632–2641.
14. Wadhwa J, Szydlo RM, Apperley JF, et al. Factors impacting on duration of survival after onset of blastic transformation of chronic myeloid leukemia. Blood 2002; 99:2304–2309.
15. O'Brien SG, Guilhot F, Larson RA, et al. Imatinib compared with interferon and low-dose cytarabine for newly diagnosed chronic-phase chronic myeloid leukemia. N Engl J Med 2003; 348:994–1004.

16. Sokal JE, Cox EB, Baccarani M, et al. and the Italian Cooperative CML Study Group. Prognostic discrimination in 'good risk' chronic granulocytic leukemia. Blood 1984; 63:789–799.

17. Druker BJ, Guilhot F, O'Brien SG, et al. Five-year follow-up of imatinib therapy for newly diagnosed chronic myeloid leukemia in chronic-phase shows sustained responses and high overall survival. N Engl J Med. In press.

18. Kantarjian H, O'Brien S, Cortes J, et al. Survival advantage with imatinib mesylate therapy in chronic-phase chronic myelogenous leukemia (CML-CP) after IFN-failure and in late CML-CP, comparison with historical controls. Clin Cancer Research 2004; 10:68–75.

19. Marin D, Marktel S, Szydlo R, et al. Survival of patients with chronic-phase chronic myeloid leukaemia on imatinib after failure of interferon alfa. Lancet 2003; 362:617–619.

20. Kantarjian H, O'Brien S, Cortes J, et al. Imatinib mesylate therapy improves survival in patients with newly diagnosed Philadelphia chromosome-positive chronic myelogenous leukemia in chronic phase. Comparison with historical data. Cancer 2003; 98:2636–2642.

21. Kantarjian H, Talpaz M, O'Brien S, et al. Survival benefit with imatinib mesylate versusinterferon alfa-based regimens in newly diagnosed chronic phase chronic myelogenous leukemia. Blood Pre-published on line May 18, 2006.

22. Roy L, Guilhot J, Krahnke T, et al. Survival advantage with imatinib compared to the combination interferon-a plus cytarabine in chronic phase CML: historical comparison between two phase III trials. Blood. Pre-published on line April 20, 2006.

23. Hasford J, Pfirrmann M, Hehlmann R, et al. A new prognostic score for survival of patients with chronic myeloid leukemia treated with interferon alfa. Writing Committee of the Collaborative CML Prognostic Factors Project Group. J Natl Cancer Inst 1998; 90:850–858.

24. Goldman JM, Lu D.-P. Chronic granulocytic leukemia—origin, prognosis and treatment. Semin Hemat 1982; 19:241–256.

25. Gordon MY, Marley SB, Apperley JF, et al. Clinical heterogeneity in chronic myeloid leukaemia reflecting biological diversity in normal persons. Br J Haematol 2003; 122:424–429.

26. Sokal JE: Prognosis in chronic myeloid leukaemia: biology of the disease vs. treatment. Baillieres Clin Haematol 1987; 1:907–929.

27. Sinclair PB, Nacheva EP, Leversha M, et al. Large deletions at the t(9;22) breakpoint are common and may identify a poor-prognosis subgroup of patients with chronic myeloid leukemia. Blood 2000; 95:738–743.

28. Huntly BJ, Reid AG, Bench AJ, et al. Deletions of the derivative chromosome 9 occur at the time of the Philadelphia translocation and provide a powerful and independent prognostic indicator in chronic myeloid leukemia. Blood 2001; 98:1732–1738.

29. Huntly BJ, Guilhot F, Reid AG, et al. Imatinib improves but may not fully reverse the poor prognosis of patients with CML with derivative chromosome 9 deletions. Blood 2003; 102:2205–2212.

30. Quintas-Cardama A, Kantarjian H, Talpaz M, et al. Imatinib mesylate therapy may overcome the poor prognostic significance of deletions of derivative chromosome 9 in patients with chronic myelogenous leukemia. Blood 2005; 105:2281–2286.

31. Yong ASM, Szydlo RM, Goldman JM, et al. Molecular profiling of CD34+ cells identifies low expression of CD7 along with high expression of proteinase 3 and elastase as predictors of longer survival in patients with CML. Blood 2006; 107:205–212.

32. Ohmine K, Ota J, Ueda M, et al. Characterization of stage progression in chronic myeloid leukemia by DNA microarray with purified hematopoietic stem cells. Oncogene 2001; 20:8249–8257.

33. Kaneta Y, Kagami Y, Katagiri T, et al. Prediction of sensitivity to STI571 among chronic myeloid leukemia patients by genome-wide cDNA microarray analysis. Jpn J Cancer Res 2002; 93:849–856.

34. Nowicki MO, Pawlowski P, Fischer T, et al. Chronic myelogenous leukemia molecular signature. Oncogene 2003; 22:3952–3963.

35. Radich J, Dai HD, Mao M, et al. Gene expression changes associated with progression and response in chronic myeloid leukemia. Proc Nat Acad Sci USA 2006; 103:2794–2799.
36. Crossman LC, Mori M, Hsieh YC, et al. In chronic myeloid leukemia white cells from cytogenetic responders and non-responders to imatinib have very similar gene expression signatures. Haematologica 2005;90:459-464.
37. White D, Saunders V, Lyons AB, et al. In-vitro sensitivity to imatinib-induced inhibition of ABL kinase activity is predictive of molecular response in de-novo CML patients. Blood 2005; 106:2520–2526.
38. Mahon FX, Belloc F, Lagarde V, et al. MDR1 gene overexpression confers resistance to imatinib mesylate in leukemia cell line models. Blood 2003; 101:2368–2373.
39. Schultheis B, Szydlo R, Mahon FX, Apperley JF, Melo JV. Analysis of total phospho-tyrosine levels in CD34+ cells from CML patients to predict the response to imatinib mesylate treatment. Blood 2005; 105:4893–4894.
40. Mahon F.-X, Belloc F, Cholet C, et al. Detection of resistance to STI571 in patients with BCR-ABL positive acute leukemia and chronic myeloid leukemia blast crisis (abstract). Blood 2000; 96:471a.
41. Jordanides NE, Jorgensen HG, Holyoake TL, Mountford JC. Functional ABCG2 is over-expressed on primary CML CD34+ cells and is inhibited by imatinib mesylate. Blood. Prepublished on line April 20, 2006.
42. Thomas J, Wang L, Clark RE, Pirmohamed M. Active transport of imatinib into and out of cells: implications for drug resistance. Blood 2004; 104:3739–3745.
43. Crossman LC, Druker BJ, Deininger MWN. hOCT1 and resistance to imatinib. Blood 2005; 106:1133–1134.
44. White DL, Saunders VA, Dang P, et al. OCT-1 mediated influx is a key determinant of the intracellular uptake of imatinib but not nilotinib (AMN107); reduced OCT-1 activity is the cause of low in vitro sensitivity to imatinib. Blood. Prepublished on line April 4, 2006.
45. Goldman JM, Marin D. Management decisions in chronic myeloid leukemia. Semin Hematol 2003; 40:97–103.
46. Baccarani M, Saglio G, Goldman JM, et al. Evolving concepts in the management of chronic myeloid leukemia. Recommendations from an expert panel on behalf of the European Leukemia-net. Blood. Prepublished on line. May 18, 2006.
47. Druker BJ, Gathmann I, Bolton A, et al. Probability and impact of obtaining a complete cytogenetic response to imatinib as initial therapy for chronic myeloid leukemia (CML) in chronic phase (abstract). Blood 2003; 102:182a.
48. Marin D, Kaeda J, Szydlo R, et al. Monitoring patients in complete cytogenetic remission after treatment of CML in chronic phase with imatinib: patterns of residual disease and prognostic factors for cytogenetic relapse. Leukemia 2005; 19:507–512.
49. Goldman JM, Gordon MY. Why do stem CML cells survive allogeneic stem cell trans-plantation or imatinib? Does it really matter? Leukemia and Lymphoma 2006; 47:1–8 (Review).
50. Holyoake T, Jiang X, Eaves C, Eaves A. Isolation of a highly quiescent subpopulation of primitive leukemic cells in chronic myeloid leukemia. Blood 1999; 94:2056–2064.
51. Graham SM, Jorgensen HG, Allan E, et al. Primitive, quiescent, Philadelphia-positive stem cells from patients with chronic myeloid leukemia are insensitive to STI571 in vitro. Blood 2002; 99:319–325.
52. Bhatia R, Holtz M, Niu N, et al. Persistence of malignant hematopoietic progenitors in chronic myelogenous leukemia patients in complete cytogenetic remission following imatinib mesylate therapy. Blood 2003; 101:4701–4707.
53. Avery S, Nadal E, Marin D, et al. Lymphoid transformation in a CML patient in complete cytogenetic remission following treatment with imatinib. Leuk Res 2004; 28(suppl): S75-S77.
54. Jabbour E, Kantarjian H, O'Brien S, et al. Sudden blastic transformation in patients with chronic myeloid leukemia treated with imatinib mesylate. Blood 2006; 107:480–482.
55. Cortes J, O'Brien S, Kantarjian H. Discontinuation of imatinib therapy after achieving a molecular response. Blood 2004; 104:2204–2205.

56. Merante S, Orlandi E, Bernasconi P, et al. Outcome for four patients with chronic myeloid leukemia after imatinib mesylate discontinuation. Haematologica 2005; 90:979–981.

57. Rousselot P, Huguet F, Rea D, et al. Imatinib mesylate discontinuation in patients with chronic myelogenous leukemia in complete molecular remission for more than two years. Blood. In press.

58. Drummond MW, Martin D, Clark RE, et al. Mobilization of Ph chromosome-negative peripheral blood stem cells in chronic myeloid leukaemia patients with imatinib mesylate-induced complete cytogenetic remission. Brit J Haematol 2003; 123:479–483.

59. Bocchia M, Gentili S, Abruzzese E, et al. Effect of p210 multipeptide vaccine with imatinib or interferon in patients with chronic myeloid leukaemia and persistent residual disease: a multicenter observational trial. Lancet 2005; 365:657–662.

60. Rojas JM, Knight K, Wang L, et al. Clinical evaluation of BCR-ABL peptide immunization in chronic myeloid leukemia: results of the EPIC study. Submitted for publication.

61. Oka Y, Tsuboi A, Taguchi T, et al. Induction of WT1 (Wilms tumor gene)-specific cytotoxic T lymphocytes by WT1 peptide vaccine and the resultant cancer regression. Proc Natl Acad Sci USA 2004; 101:13,885–13,890.

62. Molldrem JJ, Lee PP, Wang C, et al. Evidence that specific T lymphocytes may participate in the elimination of chronic myelogenous leukemia. Nat Med 2000; 6:1018–1023.

63. Smith B, Kasamon YL, Miller CB, et al. K562/GM-CSF vaccination reduces tumor burden including achieving complete molecular remissions in chronic myeloid leukemia (CML) patients (PTS) with residual disease on imatinib mesylate (IM). J Clin Oncol 2006; 24(suppl 18S):339s (Abstract #6509).

64. Olavarria E, Craddock C, Dazzi F, et al. Imatinib mesylate (STI571) in the treatment of relapse of chronic myeloid leukemia after allogeneic stem cell transplantation. Blood 2002; 99:3861–3862.

65. Kantarjian HM, O'Brien S, Cortes JE, et al. Imatinib mesylate therapy for relapse after allogeneic stem cell transplantation for chronic myelogenous leukemia. Blood 2002; 100:1590–1595.

66. Cortes J, Kantarjian H. New targeted approaches in chronic myeloid leukemia. J Clin Oncol 2005; 23:6316–6324.

67. Baccarani M, Martinelli G, Rosti G, et al. Imatinib and pegylated human recombinant interferon-alpha2b in early chronic phase chronic myeloid leukemia. Blood 2004; 104:4243–4251.

68. Gardembas M, Rousselot P, Tulliez M, et al. Results of a prospective phase 2 study combining imatinib and cytarabine for the treatment of Philadelphia-positive patients with chronic myeloid leukemia in chronic phase. Blood 2003; 4298–4305.

69. Issa J.-P, Gharibyan V, Cortes J, et al. Phase II study of low-dose decitabine in patients with chronic myelogenous leukemia resistant to imatinib mesylate. J Clin Oncol 2005; 23:3948–3956.

70. Hoover RR, Mahon FX, Melo JV, Daley QG. Overcoming STI resistance with with transferyl transferase inhibitor SCH66336. Blood 2002; 1068–1071.

71. Cortes J, Albitar M, Thomas D, et al. Efficacy of the farnesyl transferase inhibitor R115777 in chronic myeloid leukemia and other hematologic malignancies. Blood 2003; 101:1692–1697.

72. Marin D, Kaeda J, Andreasson C, et al. Phase I/II trial of adding semisynthetic homoharringtonine in chronic myeloid leukemia patients who have achieved partial or complete cytogenetic response on imatinib. Cancer 2005; 103:1850–1855.

73. Chen Y, Fan H, Pan X, et al. Coordination of intrinsic, extrinsic and endoplasmic reticulum-mediated apoptosis by imatinib mesylate combined with arsenic trioxide in chronic myeloid leukemia. Blood 2006; 107:1582–1590.

74. Marin D, Marktel S, Bua M, et al. The use of imatinib (STI571) in chronic myeloid leukemia: some practical considerations. Haematologica 2002; 87:979–988.

75. Deininger MWN, O'Brien SG, Ford JM, Druker BJ. Practical management of patients with chronic myeloid leukemia receiving imatinib. J Clin Oncol 2003; 21:1637–1647.

76. Sneed TB, Kantarjian HM, Talpaz M, et al. The significance of myelosuppression during therapy with imatinib mesylate in patients with chronic myelogenous leukemia in chronic phase. Cancer 2004; 100:116–121.
77. Guilhot F. Indications for imatinib mesylate therapy and clinical management. The Oncologist 2004; 9:271–281.
78. Ohyashiki K, Kuriyama Y, Nakajima A, et al. Imatinib mesylate induced hepato-toxicity in chronic myeloid leukemia demonstrated by focal necrosis resembling acute viral hepatitis. Leukemia 2002; 16:2160–2161.
79. Ebnoether M, Stentoft J, Ford J, et al. Cerebral oedema as a possible complication of treatment with iomatinib. Lancet 2002; 359:1751–1752.
80. Goldman JM, Druker BJ. Chronic myeloid leukemia: current treatment options. Blood 2001; 98:2039–2042.
81. Thomas DA, Faderl S, Cortes J, et al. Treatment of Philadelphia chromosome-positive acute lymphoblastic leukemia with hyper-CVAD and imatinib mesylkate. Blood 2004; 103:4396–4407.
82. Wassmann B, Pfeifer H, Goekbuget N, et al. Alternating versus concurrent schedules of imatinib and chemotherapy as front-line therapy for Philadelphia positive acute lymphoblastic leukemia (Ph + ALL). Blood. Pre-published on line April 25, 2006.

4 Monitoring Chronic Myeloid Leukemia in 2006

Nicola Hurst, Timothy P. Hughes, and Susan Branford
Institute of Medical and Veterinary Science, Adelaide, South Australia

INTRODUCTION

Chronic myeloid leukemia (CML) is well suited to molecular monitoring as rising and falling levels of BCR-ABL transcript, measured by RQ-PCR (real time quantitative polymerase chain reaction) from venous peripheral blood (PB) correlate well with disease progression and remission (1). Fluorescence in situ hybridization (FISH) and classical cytogenetics performed on bone marrow (BM) may have a role (2,3) but neither are as sensitive and reproducible for disease monitoring as RQ-PCR, especially when RQ-PCR is performed within a standardized laboratory with an optimized system(4).

The development of the tyrosine kinase inhibitor imatinib has significantly altered the management of CML with far fewer patients currently exposed to the toxicities of chemotherapy or the hazards of stem-cell transplantation. However resistance to imatinib is well documented, particularly in patients who commence imatinib in the advanced phases and may indicate a need for therapy change (1,5–10). The major mechanism of resistance is mutation within the BCR-ABL kinase domain. A greater than two-fold rising level of BCR-ABL transcript has been shown to be associated with the detection of mutations (1). This chapter will discuss molecular monitoring in the imatinib era, focusing on treatment that began in early chronic phase disease.

BCR-ABL MONITORING—A UNIQUE MARKER OF DISEASE ACTIVITY

The discovery of the Philadelphia (Ph) chromosome (11) and its molecular counterpart, the BCR-ABL fusion gene, gave CML a unique genetic marker of malignancy and, since then, much has been established about its role in cell physiology, signal transduction, and the regulation of hematopoiesis. After allogeneic BM transplant the detection of the BCR-ABL oncogene in patients with CML is significantly associated with disease relapse compared with patients in whom BCR-ABL is either not detectable or who have significantly reduced levels of transcript (12). Patients treated with interferon alpha who achieved CCyR, had prolonged disease remissions if they had undetectable levels of transcript or significantly reduced levels of transcript, compared to patients without significantly reduced levels of transcript (13). This correlation is also seen in imatinib therapy where a reduction in measurable BCR-ABL to the level of a major molecular response (MMR) is associated with a lack of disease progression, first documented in the IRIS trial (14). Table 1 defines treatment response as determined by cytogenetic and molecular analysis.

TABLE 1 Defining Response: Levels of Detectable Disease Using Different Methods and Correlation with *BCR-ABL* Ratio According to the Proposed International Scale

Level of response	Definition	Equivalent *BCR-ABL* ratio
Diagnosis in chronic phase	Peripheral blood: leucocytosis, peaks of myelocytes and neutrophils, blasts generally <2% basophils <20%, platelets normal or increased. Bone marrow blasts <5%	Range 30–300%
Complete hematological response (CHR)	Platelet <450 × 10^9 Wcc <10 × 10^9 Differential without immature granulocytes and with <5% basophils. Non palpable spleen.	
Minimal cytogenetic response	66–95% Ph positive metaphases	
Minor cytogenetic response	36–65% Ph positive metaphases	
Partial cytogenetic response (PCyR)	1–35% Ph positive metaphases	
Major cytogenetic response (MCyR)	0–35% Ph positive metaphases	10%
Complete cytogenetic response (CCyR)	0% Ph positive metaphases	1%
Major molecular response (MMR)	≥3 log reduction *BCR-ABL* mRNA from a standardized baseline	0.1%
Complete molecular response (CMR)	Undetectable *BCR-ABL* mRNA by RT-PCR at a defined level of sensitivity	0%

Source: From Ref. 4.

CYTOGENETICS AND THE DIMINISHING ROLE OF BONE MARROW ANALYSIS

The standard method for the diagnosis of CML is cytogenetic analysis, an especially useful method for demonstrating karyotypic abnormalities in addition to the Ph chromosome (clonal evolution). At diagnosis, 95% of patients have a detectable Ph chromosome, however, around one-half of patients without a detectable Ph chromosome have a demonstrable *BCR-ABL* gene. This indicates a submicroscopic insertion of *ABL* into *BCR* on chromosome 22, or *BCR* into *ABL* on chromosome 9, which is undetectable by cytogenetic analysis. Treatment response is evaluated by evidence of rising or falling numbers of cells containing the Ph chromosome using this technique of karyotype analysis. The sensitivity of the technique is limited by only 20 to 50 cells in metaphase being examined per sample. A cytogenetic abnormality may not be detected unless it is present in 2% to 5% of cells. As PB contains very few cycling myeloid cells in patients in hematological remission, BM is required for the analysis of dividing cells. This is invasive and limits the frequency of monitoring. Cells from patients treated with interferon or collected early after transplantation often fail to grow well in culture or the cell counts are low, resulting in a significant failure rate of cytogenetic analysis (3). Patients with a CCyR may still have a considerable leukemic load (15).

With accurate and reliable RQ-PCR the role of routine classical cytogenetics has lessened considerably. Regular RQ-PCR monitoring with cytogenetic analysis targeted only to patients who have not achieved or have lost MMR has been shown to represent a rational approach to monitoring, and spares most patients the discomfort of multiple marrow aspirates (16). In a study of 828 simultaneous RQ-PCR and BM cytogenetic analyses from 183 patients with chronic phase CML treated with imatinib, patients were followed for a median of 12 months. Cytogenetic progression was defined as Ph positive clonal evolution, loss of CCyR, or an increase of $\geq 20\%$ Ph-positive cells. Cytogenetic progression occurred in 24/183 (13%) patients. At the time of cytogenetic progression, none of the 24 patients had an MMR. There were 320 RQ-PCR results from 95 patients indicating MMR. No abnormality was detected in any of the corresponding cytogenetic analyses. This approach requires an accurate, reproducible RQ-PCR assay with ongoing quality assurance. Some groups have suggested that once CCyR is obtained only annual bone marrow biopsy is required (17,18). This is for the detection of myelodysplasia and clonal evolution in pH-negative cells.

FLUORESCENCE IN SITU HYBRIDIZATION

FISH uses fluorescent probes of different colors that hybridize to specific areas of DNA. The technique has a short turn-around time and generally examines ten times the number of cells routinely analyzed by cytogenetics. It can be applied to interphase or metaphase nuclei, and it has detected the *BCR-ABL* gene in patients in whom the Ph chromosome is not detectable with the help of cytogenetics. The application of the technique to interphase nuclei allows for the examination of PB so that BM sampling may not be required. However, PB may have a higher proportion of Ph negative myeloid progenitors, resulting in a lower signal compared with BM (19). The first generation of FISH probes for the detection of the Ph chromosome were single fusion with a separate colored probe for each of the *BCR* and *ABL* genes. False positive rates occurred as, by random chance, probes overlap creating a false fusion, with some laboratories reporting false positives as high as 15% (20). CML probes are now commonly dual fusion sets which span the breakpoint, leaving a residual signal on the derivative 9q proximally and extending the signal on the derivative 22q below the break. The probes hybridizing to *ABL* and *BCR* are larger and create a second fusion signal on the derivative 9q with the resulting abnormal pattern occurring very rarely as a false positive. Sensitivity is greatly improved and reliant on the number of cells that are counted (22). In a minority of patients treated with IFNα or imatinib, BM FISH may give lower Ph positive values than cytogenetic analysis (22,23). Hypermetaphase FISH involves placing 500+ cells in colchicine, a mitotic arresting agent, which allows additional chromosomal analyses to be conducted during a single collection. It can be used to detect minimal residual disease in patients in cytogenetic remission, but is not as sensitive as RQ-PCR and requires cells to be in metaphase (2).

QUANTITATIVE RT-PCR (RQ-PCR)

Quantitative RT-PCR assays for the measurement of *BCR-ABL* transcript levels in both PB and BM allow for residual disease levels to be monitored over time, providing an extremely reliable alternative for disease monitoring (12,24–35). The transcript level correlates well with the disease load present in the blood and marrow and is an accurate measure of the response to the therapy. The leukemia specific *BCR-ABL* transcript is a well-suited target for molecular monitoring as nearly all patients with CML have one of two transcript types eliminating the requirement for patient specific primers.

A variety of RQ-PCR techniques are in use that use different instruments and real time chemistry, primer and probe location, and control gene (24,25,27,28,33–37), which have differences in sensitivity and measurement reliability. It is essential that each laboratory establishes these limits for their method to allow accurate interpretation of serial monitoring. Furthermore, a series of recommendations for producing reliable data and reporting *BCR-ABL* values on an international scale have recently been published (4). These initiatives are aimed at international harmonization of RQ-PCR data.

BCR-ABL quantification by RQ-PCR has proven clinical usefulness. Imatinib-treated patients show a strong correlation between the percentage of Ph positive metaphases in the BM and the simultaneous study of PB *BCR-ABL* levels when measured by RQ-PCR (30,37,38). Early reduction of *BCR-ABL* transcript levels predicts cytogenetic response in imatinib treated chronic phase CML patients and this reduction of *BCR-ABL* is correlated with prognosis (26,32,38).

INTERNATIONAL RANDOMIZED STUDY OF INTERFERON VERSUS STI571 STUDY

The International Randomized Study of Interferon versus STI571 (IRIS) study established the superiority of 400 mg of imatinib daily over interferon and low dose cytosine arabinoside (LDAC) in a prospective randomized study of 1106 chronic phase patients (39). The rates of hematologic and cytogenetic responses were higher amongst patients with newly diagnosed chronic phase CML treated with imatinib compared with those who were treated with interferon plus cytarabine. After 12 months of treatment, molecular analysis demonstrated that an estimated 40% of patients in the imatinib group achieved a MMR, in comparison with 2% of patients in the group given interferon and LDAC (14). The frequency of achieving a MMR was highest at 50% amongst patients with low Sokal risk scores. Patients in the imatinib group who achieved a MMR had a 100% probability of remaining progression free after 24 months, compared with 95% in patients with a CCyR of <3 log reduction and 85% of patients who did not have CCyR.

After 54 months since randomization, progression free survival (PFS) in patients with a MMR was 97% compared with 89% of patients in CCyR but without a MMR and 72% in those not in CCyR. After one year 53% of patients in CCyR had achieved a MMR, however after four years 80% of these patients in CCyR had achieved a MMR. Additionally, the percentage of patients with a ≥ 4 log reduction increased from 22% to 41% (40). In patients who achieve a MMR after 12 months, transformation free survival was 100% after 54 months compared with 95% for patients in CCyR but not in MMR and 91% for patients not in CCyR after 12 months ($p = 0.0013$) (41).

After a median of 19 months of 400 mg imatinib only 3% of patients had undetectable *BCR-ABL*, at a sensitivity of 4.5 logs below the standardized baseline (14). In a separate study the percentage of patients with undetectable *BCR-ABL* was higher with longer periods of therapy and with a higher dose of imatinib (42). This proportion of patients is still low compared to patients after allogeneic hematopoietic stem-cell transplantation, where most patients have undetectable levels of *BCR-ABL* transcripts (36,43). A small population of quiescent stem cells exist that may have higher levels of *BCR-ABL* transcripts, and exhibit innate insensitivity to imatinib. These may be the leukemic cells that persist after therapy even after a complete molecular response is achieved. It has been proposed that, these cells explain molecular disease persistence and relapse and are the source of clones with kinase domain mutations (44).

IMATINIB FAILURE, SUBOPTIMAL RESPONSE, AND WARNINGS—RECOGNIZING THE NEED FOR A CHANGE IN THERAPEUTIC STRATEGY

Resistance has been previously defined as primary or secondary. Primary resistance can be defined as failure to achieve CHR by three months or MCyR by twelve months. It is not currently known what causes primary resistance. It is rarely, if indeed ever, caused by point mutations. By contrast, point mutations are the cause of 35% to 90% of cases of acquired or secondary resistance (1,5–9,45,48) Secondary resistance can be defined as progression to blast phase, progression to accelerated phase, loss of hematological response, loss of MCyR, or loss of CCyR with a ten-fold rise in *BCR-ABL* (49). Other mechanisms include drug efflux by multiresistance drug pumps (50) and gene amplification (6,8,51).

Recent recommendations from an expert panel on behalf of the European LeukemiaNet suggest criteria for determining whether treatment response is adequate at a particular treatment time point and whether a change in therapy should be considered (18). They propose to define treatment response at different time points as "failure" and "suboptimal." "Failure" means that continuing imatinib treatment at the current dose is no longer appropriate for these patients, who would likely have greater benefit from another treatment. "Suboptimal response" means the patient may still have substantial benefit from continuing imatinib, but that the long-term outcome of the treatment would not likely be as favorable as expected. Factors, which should "warn" that standard dose imatinib might not be the best choice in therapy have also been proposed, and, should these factors arise, more careful monitoring will be required.

INTERPRETING A RISING LEVEL OF *BCR-ABL* TRANSCRIPT—DETECTION AND SIGNIFICANCE OF EMERGING MUTATIONS AND IMATINIB RESISTANCE

It is postulated that mutations within the kinase domain can prevent imatinib binding by either interrupting critical contact points between imatinib and the protein or inducing a conformation to which imatinib is unable to bind (51). Imatinib binds the inactive form of the Abl kinase and functions as a competitive inhibitor of adenosine triphosphate (ATP) (52). The principle effect of imatinib binding is to block the autophosphorylation of the kinase as well as phosphorylation of key substrates so that constitutive activation of the kinase and signal transduction no longer occurs. In the presence of imatinib, Bcr-Abl is acted upon by phosphatases to remain in a predominantly unphosphorylated and enzymatically inert state. Imatinib also binds and blocks kinase activity of Pdgfr, Kit, and Fms.

An evaluation of 144 patients treated with imatinib for *BCR-ABL* kinase domain mutations by direct sequencing included 40 accelerated phase (AP), 64 late chronic phase (LCP) (defined as greater than 12 months from diagnosis), and 40 early chronic phase (ECP) patients (46). Mutations were detected in 27 patients; 33% in AP, 22% of 64 in LCP, and 0% in ECP. Acquired resistance was evident in 89% of patients with mutations. Ninety-two percent of patients with a mutation in the P-loop died with a median survival of 4.5 months, after the mutation was detected. In contrast, only 21% of patients with mutations outside the P-loop died with a median follow up of 11 months. As the detection of mutations was strongly associated with imatinib resistance, analysis was done for features that predicted their detection. Patients commencing imatinib greater than four years from diagnosis had a significantly higher incidence of mutations at 41% compared with those treated within four years at 9%. Lack of MCyR was also associated with a higher likelihood of detecting a mutation; 38% of patients without a MCyR had mutations compared with 8.5% of those with a MCyR. The detection of mutations using a direct sequencing technique was almost always associated with imatinib resistance and patients with mutations in the P-loop had a particularly poor prognosis. This finding has been supported by a number of studies, (9,10,47) although one study did not find this association (53).

The extent of resistance to imatinib conferred by different mutations varies considerably (54). The T315I mutation is highly resistant to all currently known tyrosine kinase and Src kinase inhibitors (55). Mutations outside the P-loop often respond to increased doses of imatinib whilst the detection of P-loop mutations may require a change in therapy (1,46).

The early detection of mutations should provide clinical benefit by allowing early intervention. A significant rise in the BCR-ABL level constitutes a rational basis for screening patients for mutations (1). BCR-ABL transcript levels as measured by RQ-PCR were correlated with mutation analysis in 214 patients treated with imatinib. It was determined whether there was a difference in the incidence of mutations between the patients with a more than two-fold rise in BCR-ABL and patients with stable or decreasing levels. The RQ-PCR method used in this study had measurement reliability such that a two-fold change in BCR-ABL values represented a true change at the level of a MMR rather than assay variability. Of the 56 patients with a more than two-fold rise, 34 (61%) had detectable mutations (median rise, 3.0 fold; 25th–75th percentiles, 2.3–5.2). In 31 (91%) of these 34 patients, the mutation was present at the time of the rise and became detectable within three months in the remaining patients. Only one (0.6%) of 158 patients with stable or decreasing BCR-ABL levels had a detectable mutation, $p < 0.0001$. Thus, a more than two-fold rise identified 34 (97%) of 35 patients with a mutation. The conclusion was drawn that a rise in BCR-ABL of more than two-fold can be used as a primary indicator to test patients for BCR-ABL kinase domain mutations. It is important that the measurement reliability of an RQ-PCR assay be determined so that a rise of biological significance is distinguished from assay variability (4). It is also important to note that the more than two-fold rise is not measured logarithmically, but is a linear change, (e.g., a change from 0.1% to 0.3% is a greater than two-fold rise). In our laboratory, mutation analysis is now initiated in chronic phase patients upon a significant rise in the BCR-ABL level. If a mutation is detected, the previous samples are tested to determine when the mutation first became detectable.

CASE STUDIES ILLUSTRATING THE VALUE OF MOLECULAR MONITORING

Figure 1 demonstrates the importance of monitoring patients by reliable and reproducible RQ-PCR for detecting biologically significant changes. Patient A commenced imatinib 400 mg daily in chronic phase and achieved a CCyR. A more than two-fold rise in BCR-ABL prompted mutation analysis and the non P-loop F317L mutation was identified. This mutation confers moderate resistance to imatinib. The imatinib dose was increased to 600 mg daily and the patient again achieved a sustained CCyR. Patient B commenced imatinib with a fluctuating

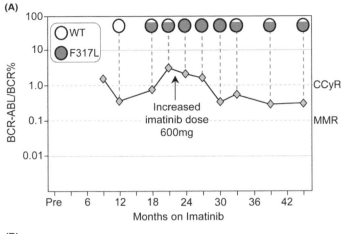

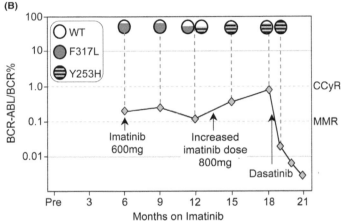

FIGURE 1 Patient response to non P-loop versus P-loop mutations. The graphs plot the *BCR-ABL* levels over the course of therapy (diamonds) and the circles represent time points of mutation analysis. The amount of shading in the circles indicates the relative amount of mutant detected compared with wild type. The proportion of imatinib sensitive non P-loop mutation is represented by block color filling in the circle while the imatinib insensitive P-loop mutation is represented by stripes.

dose of 400 to 600 mg. Molecular analysis was not performed until six months and it is unknown if a significant rise in *BCR-ABL* level occurred prior to detection of the F317L mutation. The imatinib dose was increased to 800 mg. The highly imatinib resistant P-loop mutation Y253H became detectable and the *BCR-ABL* level began to rise over the following six months. The Y253H mutation is known to be sensitive to dasatinib (56) and a MMR was achieved after dasatinib was commenced. This case illustrates the capacity of regular RQ-PCR coupled with mutation analysis to follow the complex dynamics of competing mutant clones. With this knowledge it is possible to make informed decisions about the most appropriate therapeutic response.

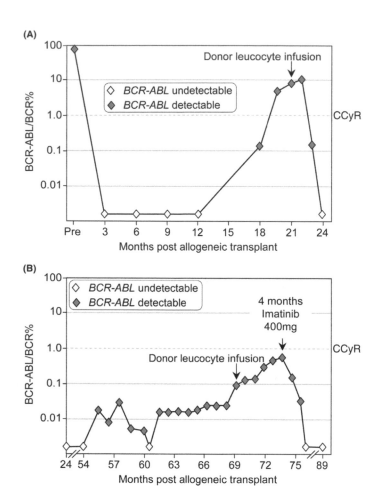

FIGURE 2 Use of molecular monitoring after allogeneic transplantation. The open diamonds represent when *BCR-ABL* is undetectable, while the black color diamonds represent when *BCR-ABL* is detectable.

Peripheral blood RQ-PCR is also performed regularly after allogeneic BM transplant to detect early relapse. Figure 2A represents a 57-year-old male who underwent nonmyeloablative allogeneic transplant. *BCR-ABL* was undetectable until 18 months of post transplant, with simultaneous cytogenetic analysis indicating CCyR. Subsequent cytogenetic analysis one month later revealed loss of CCyR. Donor leucocyte infusion (DLI) was performed and *BCR-ABL* again became undetectable until 55 months after transplant. Figure 2B represents the same patient undergoing monthly RQ-PCR after *BCR-ABL* became detectable. CCyR was maintained. A second DLI did not stop the rise in *BCR-ABL* and imatinib was given for four months. Monthly molecular analysis has demonstrated the maintenance of undetectable *BCR-ABL* after that time. This patient had a rise in *BCR-ABL* greater than 50-fold while still maintaining CCyR, which highlights the exquisite sensitivity of molecular analysis for detecting early relapse in patients post transplant.

EXPERIMENTAL MONITORING—DETECTING VARIABLES WHICH AFFECT DRUG CONCENTRATION AND IMATINIB RESPONSE

Influx and efflux mechanisms with respect to imatinib transport may have a significant effect on the concentration of imatinib that cells are ultimately exposed to. Cells receiving a lower dose of drug may be more susceptible to treatment failure. The roles of the ABC transporters *ABCB1* (Pgp) and *ABCG2* (BCRP) in imatinib drug efflux transport are still being elucidated. The most highly studied, *ABCB1* was found to influence the intracellular concentration of imatinib in some studies (57,59) but not in others (60,61). The expression of the organic cation transporter hOCT was reported to have a major role on active imatinib influx (59).

The gene for the adaptor protein CrkL (CT10 regulator of kinase like) is located centromeric to the BCR gene on chromosome 22, encoding a protein of 38 kDa molecular weight. It has been demonstrated that tyrosine phosphorylation of CrkL (p-CrkL) occurs in cells from patients with primary CML as a direct consequence of *BCR-ABL* expression (62), with levels of p-CrkL correlating well with the level of Bcr-Abl protein. When the inhibitory concentration 50% for imatinib ($IC50^{imatinib}$) was measured in patients with de novo CML, by measuring the imatinib induced reduction of p-CrkL, there was marked variability between patients. Patients with a low $IC50^{imatinib}$ had a 36% probability of achieving a 2 log reduction in *BCR-ABL* by three months compared with only 8% of patients in the high $IC50^{imatinib}$ group (63). The $IC50^{imatinib}$ was also predictive of molecular response at 12 months, with 47% of patients in the low $IC50^{imatinib}$ group achieving a MMR and 23% in the high $IC50^{imatinib}$. This data was strongly suggestive that intrinsic sensitivity to imatinib is variable in previously untreated patients with CML, and the level of Bcr-Abl kinase inhibition achieved is critical to imatinib response.

CONCLUSION

The development of standardized, reproducible RQ-PCR for *BCR-ABL* transcript has allowed for accurate disease monitoring in CML (4). Disease can be monitored using peripheral blood for RQ-PCR, reducing the need for invasive procedures such as BM biopsy in patients with stable levels of transcript (16). A significant rise in transcript reliably indicates a need for further investigation with mutation analysis and bone marrow biopsy being indicated (1). Disease can be detected and therapy changes considered and instigated below the threshold at which cytogenetics can detect disease or relapse (Figs 1 and 2). RQ-PCR should be considered an essential modality in the optimal management of CML in the targeted therapy era.

REFERENCES

1. Branford S, Rudzki Z, Parkinson I, et al. Real-time quantitative PCR analysis can be used as a primary screen to identify patients with CML treated with imatinib who have *BCR-ABL* kinase domain mutations. Blood 2004; 104(9):2926–2932.

2. Landstrom AP, Tefferi A. Fluorescent in situ hybridization in the diagnosis, prognosis, and treatment monitoring of chronic myeloid leukemia. Leuk Lymphoma 2006; 47(3): 397–402.

3. Hughes TP, Branford S. Monitoring Disease Response. In: Melo JV, Goldman JM, eds. Myeloproliferative disorders. Hematologic Malignancies: Springer-Verlag; 2006:In Press

4. Hughes TP, Deininger MW, Hochhaus A, et al. Monitoring CML patients responding to treatment with tyrosine kinase inhibitors—Review and recommendations for 'harmonizing' current methodology for detecting BCR-ABL transcripts and kinase domain mutations and for expressing results. Blood 2006; 106:28–37.

5. Shah NP, Nicoll JM, Nagar B, et al. Multiple BCR-ABL kinase domain mutations confer polyclonal resistance to the tyrosine kinase inhibitor imatinib (STI571) in chronic phase and blast crisis chronic myeloid leukemia. Cancer Cell 2002; 2(2):117–125.

6. Gorre ME, Mohammed M, Ellwood K, et al. Clinical resistance to STI-571 cancer therapy caused by BCR-ABL gene mutation or amplification. Science 2001; 293(5531):876–880.

7. Branford S, Rudzki Z, Walsh S, et al. High frequency of point mutations clustered within the adenosine triphosphate-binding region of BCR/ABL in patients with chronic myeloid leukemia or Ph-positive acute lymphoblastic leukemia who develop imatinib (STI571) resistance. Blood 2002; 99(9):3472–3475.

8. Hochhaus A, Kreil S, Corbin AS, et al. Molecular and chromosomal mechanisms of resistance to imatinib (STI571) therapy. Leukemia 2002; 16(11):2190–2196.

9. Soverini S, Martinelli G, Rosti G, et al. ABL mutations in late chronic phase chronic myeloid leukemia patients with up-front cytogenetic resistance to imatinib are associated with a greater likelihood of progression to blast crisis and shorter survival: a study by the GIMEMA Working Party on Chronic Myeloid Leukemia. J Clin Oncol 2005; 23(18):4100–4109.

10. Nicolini FE, Corm S, Le QH, et al. Mutation status and clinical outcome of 89 imatinib mesylate-resistant chronic myelogenous leukemia patients: a retrospective analysis from the French intergroup of CML (Fi(varphi)-LMC GROUP). Leukemia 2006; 20(6): 1061–1066.

11. Nowell and Hungerford. A minute chromosome in human chronic granulocytic leukemia. Science 1960; 132, 1497.

12. Olavarria E, Kanfer E, Szydlo R, et al. Early detection of BCR-ABL transcripts by quantitative reverse transcriptase-polymerase chain reaction predicts outcome after allogeneic stem cell transplantation for chronic myeloid leukemia. Blood 2001; 97(6): 1560–1565.

13. Hochhaus A, Reiter A, Reichert S, et al. Molecular heterogeneity in complete cytogenetic responders after interferon-alpha therapy for chronic myelogenous leukemia: low levels of minimal residual disease are associated with continuing remission. Blood 2000; 95(1): 62–66.

14. Hughes TP, Kaeda J, Branford S, et al. Frequency of major molecular responses to imatinib or interferon alfa plus cytarabine in newly diagnosed chronic myeloid leukemia. N Engl J Med 2003; 349(15):1423–1432.

15. Morley A. Quantifying leukemia. N Engl J Med 1998; 339(9):627–629.

16. Ross DM, Branford S, Moore S, et al. Limited clinical value of regular bone marrow cytogenetic analysis in imatinib-treated chronic phase CML patients monitored by RQ-PCR for BCR-ABL. Leukemia 2006; 20(4):664–670.

17. Hughes T, Deininger M, Hochhaus A, et al. Monitoring CML patients responding to treatment with tyrosine kinase inhibitors: review and recommendations for harmonizing current methodology for detecting BCR-ABL transcripts and kinase domain mutations and for expressing results. Blood 2006; 108(1):28–37.

18. Baccarani M, Saglio G, Goldman J, et al. Evolving concepts in the management of chronic myeloid leukemia. Recommendations from an expert panel on behalf of the European Leukemianet. Blood 2006; 108:1809–1820.

19. Sick C, Schultheis B, Pasternak G, et al. Predominantly BCR-ABL negative myeloid precursors in interferon-alpha treated chronic myelogenous leukemia: a follow-up study of peripheral blood colony-forming cells with fluorescence in situ hybridization. Ann Hematol 2001; 80(1):9–16.

20. Gozzetti A, Le Beau MM. Fluorescence in situ hybridization: uses and limitations. Semin Hematol 2000; 37(4):320–333.
21. Dewald GW, Wyatt WA, Juneau AL, et al. Highly sensitive fluorescence in situ hybridization method to detect double BCR/ABL fusion and monitor response to therapy in chronic myeloid leukemia. Blood 1998; 91(9):3357–3365.
22. Itoh T, Tamura S, Takemoto Y, et al. A cytogenetic and fluorescence in situ hybridization evaluation of interferon-alpha in the treatment of chronic myeloid leukemia. Int J Mol Med 1999; 4(6):659–663.
23. Kaeda J, Chase A, Goldman JM. Cytogenetic and molecular monitoring of residual disease in chronic myeloid leukaemia. Acta Haematol 2002; 107(2):64–75.
24. Branford S, Hughes TP, Rudzki Z. Monitoring chronic myeloid leukaemia therapy by real-time quantitative PCR in blood is a reliable alternative to bone marrow cytogenetics. Br J Haematol 1999; 107(3):587–599.
25. Emig M, Saussele S, Wittor H, et al. Accurate and rapid analysis of residual disease in patients with CML using specific fluorescent hybridization probes for real time quantitative RT-PCR. Leukemia 1999; 13(11):1825–1832.
26. Merx K, Muller MC, Kreil S, et al. Early reduction of BCR-ABL mRNA transcript levels predicts cytogenetic response in chronic phase CML patients treated with imatinib after failure of interferon alpha. Leukemia 2002; 16(9):1579–1583.
27. Lee WI, Kantarjian H, Glassman A, et al. Quantitative measurement of BCR/abl transcripts using real-time polymerase chain reaction. Ann Oncol 2002; 13(5): 781–788.
28. Wang L, Pearson K, Pillitteri L, et al. Serial monitoring of BCR-ABL by peripheral blood real-time polymerase chain reaction predicts the marrow cytogenetic response to imatinib mesylate in chronic myeloid leukaemia. Br J Haematol 2002; 118(3): 771–777.
29. Hochhaus A. Minimal residual disease in chronic myeloid leukaemia patients. Best Pract Res Clin Haematol 2002; 15(1):159–178.
30. Kantarjian HM, Talpaz M, Cortes J, et al. Quantitative polymerase chain reaction monitoring of BCR-ABL during therapy with imatinib mesylate (STI571; gleevec) in chronic-phase chronic myelogenous leukemia. Clin Cancer Res 2003; 9(1):160–166.
31. Paschka P, Muller MC, Merx K, et al. Molecular monitoring of response to imatinib (Glivec) in CML patients pretreated with interferon alpha. Low levels of residual disease are associated with continuous remission. Leukemia 2003; 17(9):1687–1694.
32. Wang L, Pearson K, Ferguson JE, et al. The early molecular response to imatinib predicts cytogenetic and clinical outcome in chronic myeloid leukaemia. Br J Haematol 2003; 120(6):990–999.
33. Stentoft J, Pallisgaard N, Kjeldsen E, et al. Kinetics of BCR-ABL fusion transcript levels in chronic myeloid leukemia patients treated with STI571 measured by quantitative real-time polymerase chain reaction. Eur J Haematol 2001; 67(5–6):302–308.
34. Barbany G, Hagberg A, Olsson-Stromberg U, et al. Manifold-assisted reverse transcription-PCR with real-time detection for measurement of the BCR-ABL fusion transcript in chronic myeloid leukemia patients. Clin Chem 2000; 46(7):913–920.
35. Cortes J, Talpaz M, O'Brien S, et al. Molecular Responses in Patients with Chronic Myelogenous Leukemia in Chronic Phase Treated with Imatinib Mesylate. Clin Cancer Res 2005; 11(9):3425–3432.
36. Radich JP, Gooley T, Bryant E, et al. The significance of bcr-abl molecular detection in chronic myeloid leukemia patients "late," 18 months or more after transplantation. Blood 2001; 98(6):1701–1707.
37. Gabert J, Beillard E, van der Velden VH, et al. Standardization and quality control studies of 'real-time' quantitative reverse transcriptase polymerase chain reaction of fusion gene transcripts for residual disease detection in leukemia—a Europe Against Cancer program. Leukemia 2003; 17(12):2318–2357.
38. Branford S, Rudzki Z, Harper A, et al. Imatinib produces significantly superior molecular responses compared to interferon alfa plus cytarabine in patients with newly diagnosed chronic myeloid leukemia in chronic phase. Leukemia 2003; 17(12): 2401–2409.

39. O'Brien SG, Guilhot F, Larson RA, et al. Imatinib compared with interferon and low-dose cytarabine for newly diagnosed chronic-phase chronic myeloid leukemia. N Engl J Med 2003; 348(11):994–1004.
40. Goldman JM, Hughes T, Radich J, et al. Continuing reduction in level of residual disease after 4 years in patients with CML in chronic phase responding to first-line imatinib (IM) in the IRIS study. ASH Annual Meeting Abstracts. Blood 2005; 106(11):51a [abstract 163].
41. Simonsson B, On Behalf of the ISG. Beneficial effects of cytogenetic and molecular response on long-term outcome in patients with newly diagnosed Chronic Myeloid Leukemia in chronic phase (CML-CP) treated with imatinib (IM): Update from the IRIS Study. ASH Annual Meeting Abstracts. Blood 2005; 106(11):52a [abstract 166].
42. Kantarjian H, Talpaz M, O'Brien S, et al. High-dose imatinib mesylate therapy in newly diagnosed Philadelphia chromosome-positive chronic phase chronic myeloid leukemia. Blood 2004; 103(8):2873–2878.
43. Cross NC, Feng L, Chase A, et al. Competitive polymerase chain reaction to estimate the number of BCR-ABL transcripts in chronic myeloid leukemia patients after bone marrow transplantation. Blood 1993; 82(6):1929–1936.
44. Elrick LJ, Jorgensen HG, Mountford JC, et al. Punish the parent not the progeny. Blood 2005; 105(5):1862–1866.
45. Soverini S, Martinelli G, Rosti G, et al. ABL mutations in late-chronic phase chronic myeloid leukemia patients with cytogenetic refractoriness to imatinib are associated with a greater likelihood of progression to blast crisis and shorter survival. Blood 2004; 104:287a [abstract 1005].
46. Branford S, Rudzki Z, Walsh S, et al. Detection of BCR-ABL mutations in patients with CML treated with imatinib is virtually always accompanied by clinical resistance, and mutations in the ATP phosphate-binding loop (P-loop) are associated with a poor prognosis. Blood 2003; 102(1):276–283.
47. Kreil S, Mueller M, Hanfstein B, et al. Management and clinical outcome of CML patients after imatinib resistance associated with ABL kinase domain mutations [abstract]. Blood 2003; 102:71a [abstract 238].
48. Al-Ali HK, Heinrich MC, Lange T, et al. High incidence of BCR-ABL kinase domain mutations and absence of mutations of the PDGFR and KIT activation loops in CML patients with secondary resistance to imatinib. Hematol J 2004; 5(1):55–60.
49. Goldman JM. Chronic myeloid leukemia-still a few questions. Exp Hematol 2004; 32(1):2–10.
50. Mahon FX, Deininger MW, Schultheis B, et al. Selection and characterization of BCR-ABL positive cell lines with differential sensitivity to the tyrosine kinase inhibitor STI571: diverse mechanisms of resistance. Blood 2000; 96(3):1070–1079.
51. Gambacorti-Passerini CB, Gunby RH, Piazza R, et al. Molecular mechanisms of resistance to imatinib in Philadelphia-chromosome-positive leukaemias. Lancet Oncol 2003; 4(2):75–85.
52. Schindler T, Bornmann W, Pellicena P, et al. Structural mechanism for STI-571 inhibition of abelson tyrosine kinase. Science 2000; 289(5486):1938–1942.
53. Jabbour E, Kantarjian H, Jones D, et al. Long-term incidence and outcome of BCR-ABL mutations in patients (pts) with chronic myeloid leukemia (CML) treated with imatinib mesylate—P-Loop mutations are not associated with worse outcome [abstract]. ASH Annual Meeting Abstracts 2004; 104:288a.
54. O'Hare T, Walters DK, Stoffregen EP, et al. In vitro activity of Bcr-Abl inhibitors AMN107 and BMS-354825 against clinically relevant imatinib-resistant Abl kinase domain mutants. Cancer Res 2005; 65(11):4500–4505.
55. Shah NP. Loss of Response to Imatinib: Mechanisms and Management. Hematology 2005; 2005(1):183–187.
56. Shah NP, Tran C, Lee FY, et al. Overriding imatinib resistance with a novel ABL kinase inhibitor. Science 2004; 305(5682):399–401.
57. Mahon FX, Belloc F, Lagarde V, et al. MDR1 gene overexpression confers resistance to imatinib mesylate in leukemia cell line models. Blood 2003; 101(6):2368–2373.

58. Illmer T, Schaich M, Platzbecker U, et al. P-glycoprotein-mediated drug efflux is a resistance mechanism of chronic myelogenous leukemia cells to treatment with imatinib mesylate. Leukemia 2004; 18(3):401–408.
59. Thomas J, Wang L, Clark RE, et al. Active transport of imatinib into and out of cells: implications for drug resistance. Blood 2004; 104(12):3739–3745.
60. Ferrao PT, Frost MJ, Siah SP, et al. Overexpression of P-glycoprotein in K562 cells does not confer resistance to the growth inhibitory effects of imatinib (STI571) in vitro. Blood 2003; 102(13):4499–4503.
61. Zong Y, Zhou S, Sorrentino BP. Loss of P-glycoprotein expression in hematopoietic stem cells does not improve responses to imatinib in a murine model of chronic myelogenous leukemia. Leukemia 2005; 19(9):1590–1596.
62. Nichols GL, Raines MA, Vera JC, et al. Identification of CRKL as the constitutively phosphorylated 39-kD tyrosine phosphoprotein in chronic myelogenous leukemia cells. Blood 1994; 84(9):2912–2918.
63. White D, Saunders V, Lyons AB, et al. In vitro sensitivity to imatinib-induced inhibition of ABL kinase activity is predictive of molecular response in patients with de novo CML. Blood 2005; 106(7):2520–2526.

Dasatinib: A Dual ABL and SRC Inhibitor

Alfonso Quintás-Cardama, Hagop Kantarjian, and Jorge Cortes

Department of Leukemia, University of Texas M.D. Anderson Cancer Center, Houston, Texas, U.S.A.

INTRODUCTION

The hallmark of chronic myeloid leukemia (CML) is the presence of a balanced translocation, t(9;22)(q34;q11.2), known as the Philadelphia (Ph) chromosome (1,2). This juxtaposes two genes, *ABL*, which encodes a protein with tyrosine kinase activity, and *BCR*, which encodes a protein with serine kinase activity. The result is a fusion gene, *BCR-ABL*, which upon translation gives rise to a fusion protein with increased tyrosine kinase activity. Imatinib mesylate (Gleevec[TM]) has become standard therapy in CML with complete hematologic response (CHR) in 98% and complete cytogenetic response (CCyR) in 87%, with a survival free from transformation of 93% after 60 months of follow-up among patients treated in early chronic phase (CP) in the IRIS trial (3). However, a subset of patients have either primary or secondary resistance to imatinib. Several mechanisms of resistance have been identified in these patients. The most common mechanism of resistance is the development of mutations in the Abl kinase domain, but other mechanisms have been identified, including overexpression or amplification of *BCR-ABL* or its protein product, disruption of the transport of imatinib into the cells or increased transport out of the cells, and *BCR-ABL*–independent mechanisms such as the overexpression of Src-related kinases. These are described in more detail in Chapter 7. Several strategies are being investigated in order to overcome imatinib resistance, including the development of novel tyrosine kinase inhibitors with enhanced activity against Bcr-Abl compared to imatinib and/or inhibitory activity against other kinases that modulate downstream Bcr-Abl signaling pathways.

SRC: A TARGET FOR CHRONIC MYELOID LEUKEMIA THERAPY

Src kinases represent a family of nine structurally homologous nonreceptor intracellular tyrosine kinases (Src, Fyn, Yes, Blk, Yrk, Fgr, Hck, Lck, and Lyn) that regulate signal transduction pathways involved in cell growth, differentiation, and survival (4). The expression of some Src kinases is ubiquitous, whereas others display more tissue-specific patterns of expression. For example, Hck, Lyn, Fgr, Lck, and Blk are strictly restricted to hematopoietic cells (4). Furthermore, Hck is circumscribed to myeloid cells and B-lymphocytes, whereas Lyn is expressed in myeloid cells, B-lymphocytes, and NK cells (4). In addition, multiple domains of Bcr-Abl interact with Hck and Lyn leading to their activation, and experiments with Src dominant-negative mutants suggest that Src kinases play a role in proliferation of *BCR-ABL*–expressing cell lines (4–6). However, neither the formation of the Hck-Bcr-Abl complex nor the Bcr-Abl–mediated activation of Hck is dependent on the Abl kinase activity (7). Overexpression of Src family of kinases has also been implicated in *BCR-ABL*–mediated leukemogenesis and, in some cases, in imatinib resistance (8–11). Paired samples from patients with CML obtained before and after imatinib failure suggested that overexpression of Hck and Lyn occurred during CML progression to blast phase (BP), suggesting that acquired imatinib resistance may be mediated by overexpression of Src kinases in at least some patients (9). Activation of Src kinases may promote phosphorylation of *BCR-ABL* and interaction with Grb2 (6,7). In addition, Abl has significant sequence homology with Src and, in its active configuration, it bears a remarkable structural resemblance with Src family kinases. ATP-competitive compounds originally developed as Src inhibitors frequently have potent inhibition of Abl kinase due to the striking resemblance between the catalytically active state of both protein kinases (12). On the basis of the structural similarity between Abl and Src and their proposed critical role in the pathogenesis of CML, it could be hypothesized that small molecule inhibitors with activity against both *ABL* and Src may have increased activity in CML compared to that of more selective inhibitors, such as imatinib that has negligible activity against Src kinases. This may be at least partially due to the fact that in the inactive configuration, the only one to which imatinib can bind, Abl is much less structurally similar to Src.

PRECLINICAL DEVELOPMENT OF DASATINIB

A series of substituted 2-(aminopyridyl)- and 2-(aminopyrimidinyl)thiazole-5-carboxamides, initially developed as immunosuppressant drugs, were identified as potent dual Src and Abl kinase inhibitors (13). Dasatinib (BMS-354825, Sprycel™, N-(2-chloro-6-methylphenyl)-2-(6-(4-(2-hydroxyethyl)piperazin-1-yl)-2-methylpyrimidin-4-lamino) thiazole-5-carboxamide) was selected for further in vivo studies on the basis of its modest plasma protein binding and sustained blood levels in four-hour exposure studies (Fig. 1) (13). The three-dimensional crystal structure of dasatinib complexed with the Abl kinase domain revealed the presence of two hydrogen bonds at the hinge region of the ATP-binding site involving Met318, and one hydrogen bond between the hydroxyl oxygen of Thr315 and the amide nitrogen of dasatinib (13). Similar bonds occur between dasatinib and Src kinase, with the addition of another hydrogen bond between dasatinib and the Src residue Lys295 (13). Dasatinib effectively inhibited several Src family kinases, including Src (IC$_{50}$ 0.55 nM), Lck (IC$_{50}$ 1.1 nM), Fyn (IC$_{50}$ 0.2 nM), and Yes (IC$_{50}$ 0.41 nM). In addition, dasatinib demonstrated significant activity against Abl (IC$_{50}$ <1 nM), Kit (IC$_{50}$ 13 nM), Pdgfrβ (IC$_{50}$ 28 nM), and Epha2 (IC$_{50}$ 17 nM), and some activity against Her1 (IC$_{50}$ 180 nM), and p38 Map (IC$_{50}$ 100 nM) kinases (13,14). Because of its less stringent binding requirements, dasatinib binds both the active and inactive conformations of the Abl kinase. A possible

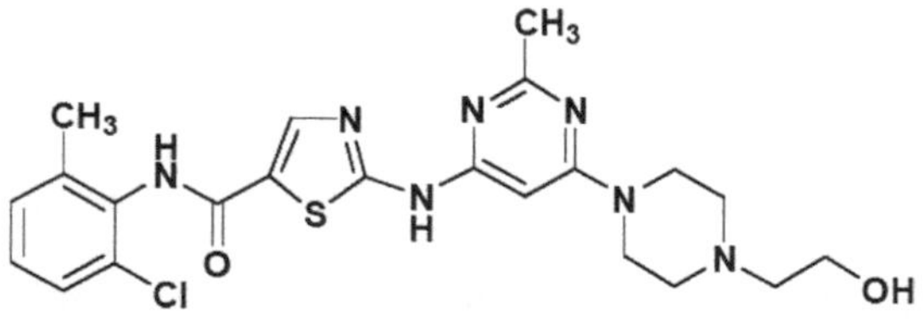

FIGURE 1 Chemical structure of dasatinib (BMS-354825).

consequence of the inhibition of the Src family kinases is that dasatinib also inhibits the proliferation of solid tumor cell lines, such as MDA-MB-211 (breast; IC_{50} 10-12 nM), PC-3 (prostate; IC_{50} 5-9 nM), WiDr (colon; IC_{50} 38-52 nM), and H69 and H526 (small cell lung cancer), in vitro and/or in tumor xenograft models. This has generated interest in investigating dasatinib for the treatment of solid tumors (13,14).

Pharmacokinetics in a rat model identified a high volume of distribution (V_{ss} 6.3 L/kg) for dasatinib with systemic clearance of approximately 40% of hepatic blood flow. A 10 mg/kg oral dose was rapidly absorbed and demonstrated a favorable half-life ($t_{1/2}$ 3.1 hours) and measured oral bioavailability of 27%. The in vivo activity of dasatinib was evaluated in a K562 xenograft model of CML, demonstrating complete tumor regressions and low toxicity at doses ranging from 5 to 50 mg/kg in a five day on, two day off schedule, without significant toxicity (13).

In cellular assays, dasatinib inhibited the proliferation of BCR-ABL–transfected Ba/F3 cells and human Bcr-Abl–expressing K562 cells with IC_{50} values of 1.3 and <1 nM, respectively, and demonstrated high potency against 14 of 15 clinically relevant imatinib-resistant Abl mutations (14–16), supporting the less stringent conformational requirements of dasatinib on Abl for kinase inhibition compared to imatinib (15). Of note, the T315I retained kinase activity even in the presence of μM concentrations of dasatinib, suggesting that this residue acts as a gate-keeper for ATP-competitive small-molecule kinase inhibitors. In a model of imatinib-resistant, BCR-ABL–mediated disease, severe combined immunodeficient (SCID) mice were injected intravenously with Ba/F3 cells expressing different Bcr-Abl isoforms as well as the firefly luciferase gene. Administration of dasatinib 10 mg/kg twice daily by oral gavage for two weeks resulted in mice showing greater than 1-log lower levels of bioluminescent activity and prolonged survival compared with untreated controls. Mice with the T315I mutation did not respond. Notably, dasatinib markedly inhibited the growth of bone marrow progenitors isolated from patients with CML with imatinib-sensitive or -resistant (M351T) disease, but not marrow progenitors obtained from healthy volunteers (15). In a saturation mutagenesis screening, significantly fewer mutations were induced with dasatinib compared to imatinib. Still, 10 Bcr-Abl mutants were generated, with the most frequent being F317V > T315A > T315I > F317L. All these mutants represent points of contact between dasatinib and the Abl kinase. These mutants could potentially account for clinical resistance to dasatinib in clinical practice. In fact, instances of dasatinib failure associated with one of these mutations, T315A, have been described (17). Interestingly, this mutation is effectively inhibited by imatinib. Of note, the combination of dasatinib with imatinib greatly reduced the recovery of drug-resistant clones (17). Similar results were observed in another cell-line based mutagenesis assay (18).

Most patients treated with imatinib have minimal residual disease as detected by polymerase chain reaction (PCR) (19). This has been associated with persistence of primitive leukemic progenitors (20). Bcr-Abl–expressing CD34+/Lin– leukemic stem cells of patients with CP CML remained viable in a quiescent state even in the presence of growth factors and imatinib (21), likely heralding relapse even after prolonged exposure to imatinib (22). Although dasatinib is significantly more potent than imatinib within the CML stem cell compartment, some quiescent stem cells survive, suggesting that this population may be innately insensitive, at least to some extent, to both agents (23). Moreover, several imatinib-resistant Abl kinase domain mutations have been detected in CD34+/BCR-ABL+ progenitors

(24), and the activity of both imatinib and dasatinib against K562 cells forced into quiescence by nutrient depletion is approximately 10-fold lower than against proliferating K562 cells (25). Interestingly, studies in quiescent K562 cultures and in murine K562 xenografts demonstrated that the combination of dasatinib with the farnesyl transferase inhibitor BMS-214662 produced supra-additive cytotoxicity at clinically achievable concentrations (25).

It has been reported that therapy with imatinib in patients with CML results in significantly lower percentages of CD4+ T cells that synthesized interleukin 2 (IL-2), interferon-γ (IFN-γ), and tumor necrosis factor-α (TNF-α) than the activated T cells of control subjects, which translates into decreased T cell proliferation in vitro (26). Noteworthy, no effects were observed on the ability of activated T cells, obtained from patients with CP CML during dasatinib treatment, to synthesize IL-2, IL-10, IFN-γ, or TNF-α cytokines despite the potent activity of dasatinib against Src family kinases (27).

CLINICAL DEVELOPMENT OF DASATINIB IN CHRONIC MYELOID LEUKEMIA

Dasatinib was first investigated in a phase I dose-escalating study involving patients with CML in all phases who had failed or developed intolerance to imatinib therapy (Table 1). Initially, dasatinib was administered only to patients with CP on a once-daily schedule for five consecutive days, followed by two days without treatment every week, and later a twice-daily administration was also investigated as well as a continuous daily administration. After clinical activity was observed in CP, patients with accelerated phase (AP) or BP and patients with Philadelphia positive acute lymphoblastic leukemia (Ph+ ALL) were included, all of them treated with the twice-daily schedule. Within two hours of oral administration of the higher doses, plasma concentrations in the range of 100 to 200 nM were achieved and a terminal half-life of about five hours was reported (28). A total of

TABLE 1 Response to Dasatinib in Patients with Chronic Myeloid Leukemia Who Have Developed Resistance or Intolerance to Imatinib

				Response (%)			
				Hematologic		Cytogenetic	
Study	Agent	CML phase	No.	Overall	Complete	Overall	Complete
Phase I	Dasatinib	CP	40	93	93	63	35
		AP	11	81	45	36	18
		MyBP	23	61	35	52	26
		LyBP	10	80	70	90	30
Phase II	Dasatinib	CP	387	90	90	51	40
		AP	174	59	34	39	25
		MyBP	109	49	25	44	25
		LyBP-Ph + ALL	94	44	31	54	40

Abbreviations: AP, accelerated phase; CE, clonal evolution; CML, chronic myeloid leukemia; CP, chronic phase; LyBP, lymphoid blast phase; Ph+ ALL, Philadelphia chromosome-positive acute lymphoblastic leukemia; MyBP, myeloid blast phase.

84 patients (40 in CP, 11 in AP, 23 in myeloid BP, and 10 with Ph+ ALL) received dasatinib 15 to 240 mg daily (29). A CHR was achieved in 37 (93%) patients in CP and a major cytogenetic response (MCyR) in 18 (45%), including a CCyR in 14 (35%). Major hematologic responses were observed in 31 (70%) of 44 patients with AP, BP, or Ph+ ALL, and MCyR were achieved in 27%, 35%, and 80% of patients in AP, BP, and Ph+ ALL, respectively. Responses were maintained in 95% of patients with CP and in 82% of patients with AP after a median follow-up of more than 12 and 5 months, respectively. However, only one (10%) patient with Ph+ ALL remained relapse-free after a median follow-up of four months (29). Overall, therapy with dasatinib therapy was well tolerated. The most frequently described toxicities were myelosuppression, gastrointestinal, and fluid retention syndromes. Grade 3–4 neutropenia or thrombocytopenia was observed in 45% and 35% of patients treated in CP and in 89% and 80% of those with AP, BP, or Ph+ ALL, respectively. Diarrhea occurred in 23% of patients, but was grade 1–2 in all but one patient. Fifteen (18%) patients had nonmalignant pleural effusions likely related to dasatinib therapy, usually grade 1 or 2 and grade 1–2 peripheral edema was observed in 16 (19%) patients. In this phase I study, 60 (71%) of 84 patients presented *BCR-ABL* mutations at baseline. CHR and cytogenetic responses were observed across all mutations, except in the four patients who had the T315I mutation, including one patient who developed this mutation while receiving dasatinib (29).

Results from a series of open-label phase II studies of dasatinib in patients with CML in all phases who had failed or become intolerant to imatinib, have been recently reported (Table 1). In these studies, dasatinib was administered at a dose of 70 mg twice daily based on pharmacokinetic data and optimal inhibition of Bcr-Abl and Src activity (28). In one study, involving exclusively patients in CP, 387 patients resistant (75%) or intolerant (25%) to imatinib with a median age of 58 years (range, 21–85 years) were treated (30). Dose escalation to 90 mg twice daily was permitted in patients achieving suboptimal response, and dose reductions down to 40 mg twice daily were allowed in those who developed intolerance. A CHR was observed in 90% of patients, and MCyR was reported in 78% of imatinib-intolerant (68% CCyR and 10% PCyR) and in 42% of imatinib-resistant (30% CCyR and 12% PCyR) patients. *BCR-ABL* mutations were detected in 160 (44%) of 363 assessable patients, with G250E ($n = 23$) being the most frequent. T315I was present in only three patients. Significant molecular responses were not observed until after six months of dasatinib therapy, with a median Bcr-Abl/Abl ratio of 0.3% at nine months (30). The 10-months progression-free survival was 88%. The most common nonhematologic toxicity was diarrhea (32%), headache (30%), rash (22%), superficial edema (20%), and pleural effusion (17%), but most of these were grade 1 or 2. Grade 3 or 4 nonhematologic toxicity included pleural effusion in 3%, and diarrhea and liver toxicity in 2% each. Neutropenia or thrombocytopenia grade 3 or 4 were reported in 47% of patients each (30).

A total of 174 patients with CML AP were treated with dasatinib in another phase II study (31). Ninety-one (52%) patients had failed imatinib therapy at doses equal or higher than 600 mg daily. Dose escalation up to 100 mg twice daily or reductions down to 40 mg twice daily were allowed for poor initial response or dasatinib-related toxicity, respectively. The median duration of dasatinib therapy was seven months (range, 0.13–13), and the average daily dasatinib dose was 113 mg (range, 24–192). Dasatinib dose was reduced in 53% and escalated in 46% of patients, respectively, and 63 (36%) patients eventually discontinued dasatinib, mainly due to disease progression ($n = 27$), toxicity ($n = 10$), or death ($n = 10$). A major hematologic response was reported in 102 (59%) patients, including 59 (34%) who achieved a CHR and 43 (25%) with no evidence of leukemia (NEL). A MCyR was attained by 60 (34%), including 43 (25%) and 17 (10%) patients who had CCyR and PCyR, respectively. MCyR occurred in 34 (36%) of 94 patients harboring Bcr-Abl mutations. The majority of patients (97%) experienced some degree of cytopenias, although 18% and 45% of patients entered the study with baseline neutropenia and thrombocytopenia, respectively. The most common nonhematologic toxicities were diarrhea (61%) and rash (27%), mostly grade 1 and 2. Grade 3 or 4 diarrhea occurred in 10%, but could be managed with proper therapy. Pleural effusion was observed in 43 (25%) patients, but it was grade 3 or 4 in only 5 (3%) and was manageable with diuretics and/or pulse steroids (31).

Preliminary data after a minimum follow-up of six months were reported in 109 patients with CML myeloid BP (32) and in 94 patients with either CML lymphoid BP ($n = 48$) or Ph+ ALL ($n = 46$) (33). Ninety-one percent of patients were resistant to imatinib in each group and the proportion of patients who had failed imatinib therapy at doses equal or higher than 600 mg daily were 50%, 52%, and 46% for patients with myeloid BP, lymphoid BP, and Ph+ ALL, respectively. Dose escalation to 100 mg twice daily or reduction to 50 and 40 mg twice daily was permitted. The overall hematologic and cytogenetic response rates among patients with myeloid BP were 49% (50% for imatinib-resistant and 40% for imatinib-intolerant) and 44% (CCyR 25%, PCyR 6%, and minor/minimal cytogenetic response 13%), respectively. Major hematologic responses were observed in 33% (CHR 29% and NEL 4%) patients with lymphoid BP and in 39% (CHR 33% and NEL 7%) among those with Ph+ ALL and MCyR were reported in 44% (CCyR 38%) of patients with lymphoid BP and in 46% (CCyR 44%) of those with Ph+ ALL. Dasatinib therapy was associated with rapid and profound myelosuppression in all groups of patients, although this was pre-existing in a substantial proportion of patients. Grade 3–4 neutropenia or thrombocytopenia was observed in 64% (18% at baseline) and 64% (43% at baseline) of patients with CML in myeloid BP and in 81%/74% (48%/20% at baseline) and 88%/78% (67%/48% at baseline) in those with lymphoid BP/Ph+ ALL, respectively. The most frequent nonhematologic toxicities included diarrhea (30–37%), nausea (18–22%), and vomiting (17–20%), which were generally grade 1–2 and manageable. Pleural effusion was observed in 30% (grade 3–4 in 13%) of patients receiving dasatinib in myeloid BP and in 16% (grade 3–4 in 4%) of patients with lymphoid BP/Ph+ ALL (32,33).

In summary, the results from the phase I and II studies demonstrate significant clinical activity of dasatinib in all stages of CML. Responses have been durable to the extent of the follow-up available to date, particularly among patients treated in CP and AP and less so in the BP. In addition, responses have been observed across a wide range of mutations, except T315I, confirming the results obtained in vitro. Dasatinib has been overall well tolerated. Myelosuppression occurs in many patients, particularly those treated in AP and BP, who start therapy with an already compromised marrow reserve. In most instances, myelosuppression is transient and rapidly reversible. Among nonhematologic adverse events, most are mild and manageable. Fluid retention has received significant attention, particularly in the form of pleural effusion. This is more common (20–30%) in BP than in earlier stages (10–15% in CP) and is frequently mild, with grade 3–4 cases present in only 3% to 5% in CP and 10% to 15% in BP. This can usually be managed with transient treatment interruptions and use of diuretics and corticosteroids. Only occasionally does it require thoracentesis, and it rarely results in permanent treatment discontinuation. Other adverse events have been usually mild and manageable.

Recently, results from a randomized, multinational, open-label phase II study comparing the activity of dasatinib and high-dose imatinib have been reported (34). The analysis was based on data from 150 imatinib-resistant patients randomized 2:1 to receive dasatinib 70 mg twice daily or imatinib 400 mg twice daily. Crossover was allowed for progression, lack of response, or intolerance. After a follow-up of three months, MCyR was achieved in 35% (CCyR 21% and PCyR 14%) of patients in the dasatinib arm and in 29% (CCyR 8% and PCyR 21%) in the high-dose imatinib arm. In addition, 15% of patients in the dasatinib arm and 76% in the imatinib arm had progression or crossover. Interestingly, among 19 patients who crossed over to dasatinib therapy, 42% achieved a MCyR while none of the four who crossed over to imatinib achieved MCyR. There were no significant differences in the toxicities between both arms, except for the occurrence of pleural effusion in 11% of patients treated with dasatinib (34).

A molecular analysis of imatinib resistant/intolerant patients (19 in CP and 14 with advanced disease (AP, BP, and Ph+ ALL) treated at UCLA in the phase I dose escalation trial of dasatinib showed that 6 (43%) of 14 patients in advanced phase and 7 (37%) of 19 in CP achieved ≥2-log reductions, including four patients in each group who had a major molecular response (MMR) as measured by quantitative polymerase chain reaction (PCR). More important, responses were maintained in two of six patients with advanced disease, and six of seven in CP achieving ≥2 log reductions. Mutations were detected at last analysis in all 23 patients with baseline mutations. The same mutation that was present at baseline was present in 21 patients and five of them had an additional mutation. Mutations were present in all patients who progressed (1 CP, 7 AP/BC) and it was T315I in six of them. T315I evolved in three other patients who have not progressed (1CP, 2 AP/BC), making this mutant the most frequently detected during dasatinib therapy, and it was accompanied by significant increase in Bcr-Abl transcripts in all patients (35).

Another analysis of the dynamics of molecular response to dasatinib has been recently reported (36). Fifty-four patients [CP = 29 (55%), AP = 14 (26%), and BP = 10 (19%)] received dasatinib at 140 mg daily ($n = 49$) or at 100 mg daily ($n = 4$) in phase II studies for a median of 36 weeks (range, 11–73). Patients in CP had a baseline median *BCR-ABL/ABL* ratio of 68.99%. After two months of therapy a significant decrease in the *BCR-ABL* transcript level was observed, with a median value of 11.64%. By nine months the median value had decreased to 0.12%. In contrast, patients with advanced phase CML (baseline *BCR-ABL/ABL* ratio of 100%) experienced a steady decline in transcript levels from the start of dasatinib therapy, but the decline was slower and less pronounced than that observed in CP. The lowest median PCR value achieved by this group of patients was observed at nine months (0.94%). At this time point, the median *BCR-ABL* transcript level reached by these patients was similar to that achieved by patients in CP at six months (0.99%). Ten patients achieved at least an MMR (*BCR-ABL/ABL* ratio below 0.05%) by quantitative real-time PCR, with three of them having undetectable *BCR-ABL* levels. All 10 patients who achieved a MMR were in CP at the start of dasatinib therapy, and three of five evaluated had an Abl kinase domain mutation at the start of the therapy. No T315I mutations were observed in this study (36).

CONCLUSION

Despite the excellent results obtained with imatinib, there is still a clear need to improve therapy in CML. The remarkable response rates obtained with dasatinib in patients with CML in the postimatinib failure setting with an acceptable toxicity profile has prompted the undertaking of several ongoing clinical trials aiming to address the activity of this dual Src/Abl inhibitor in newly diagnosed patients with CML. However, there are still important questions regarding the optimal use of dasatinib in CML, such as the correct dasatinib schedule (daily versus twice daily) and dosage (total daily dose of 100 mg versus 140 mg) that will permit to maximize cytogenetic and molecular responses with optimal tolerability and safety. Further follow-up of patients currently on dasatinib therapy will provide invaluable information that will help to accurately define the molecular response rates obtained with this agent, their durability, and dasatinib-associated long-term toxicity. Moreover, it remains uncertain whether the in vitro activity of dasatinib observed against primitive quiescent leukemic cells will translate into improved and more durable response rates in CML, particularly when used in the frontline setting. Finally, it will be particularly appealing to investigate if combinations of dasatinib with other tyrosine kinases, such as imatinib or nilotinib (AMN107), or other inhibitors, such as farnesyl transferase inhibitors, will improve upon the activity of any of these agents alone.

REFERENCES

1. Nowell P, Hungerford, D. A minute chromosome in human chronic granulocytic leukemia. Science 1960; 132:1497.
2. Rowley J. A new consistent chromosomal abnormality in chronic myelogenous leukaemia identified by quinacrine fluorescence and Giemsa staining. Nature 1973; 243:290–293.
3. Druker B, Guilhot F, O'Brien, S, et al. Long-term benefits of imatinib (IM) for patients newly diagnosed with chronic myelogenous leukemia in chronic phase (CML-CP): The 5-year update from the IRIS study. Proc Am Soc Clin Oncol 2006; 24:(abstr 6506).
4. Abram CL, Courtneidge SA. Src family tyrosine kinases and growth factor signaling. Exp Cell Res 2000; 254:1–13.
5. Stanglmaier M, Warmuth M, Kleinlein I, Reis S, Hallek M. The interaction of the Bcr-Abl tyrosine kinase with the Src kinase Hck is mediated by multiple binding domains. Leukemia 2003; 17:283–289.
6. Danhauser-Riedl S, Warmuth M, Druker BJ, Emmerich B, Hallek M. Activation of Src kinases p53/56lyn and p59hck by p210bcr/abl in myeloid cells. Cancer Res 1996; 56:3589–3596.
7. Warmuth M, Bergmann M, Priess A, Hauslmann K, Emmerich B, Hallek M. The Src family kinase Hck interacts with Bcr-Abl by a kinase-independent mechanism and phosphorylates the Grb2-binding site of Bcr. J Biol Chem 1997; 272:33,260–33,270.
8. Dai Y, Rahmani M, Corey SJ, Dent P, Grant S. A Bcr/Abl-independent, Lyn-dependent form of imatinib mesylate (STI-571) resistance is associated with altered expression of Bcl-2. J Biol Chem 2004; 279:34,227–34,239.
9. Donato NJ, Wu JY, Stapley J, et al. BCR-ABL independence and LYN kinase overexpression in chronic myelogenous leukemia cells selected for resistance to STI571. Blood 2003; 101:690–698.
10. Donato NJ, Wu JY, Stapley J, et al. Imatinib mesylate resistance through BCR-ABL independence in chronic myelogenous leukemia. Cancer Res 2004; 64:672–677.

11. Hofmann WK, Jones LC, Lemp NA, et al. Ph(+) acute lymphoblastic leukemia resistant to the tyrosine kinase inhibitor STI571 has a unique *BCR-ABL* gene mutation. Blood 2002; 99:1860–1862.

12. Nagar B, Bornmann WG, Pellicena P, et al. Crystal structures of the kinase domain of c-Abl in complex with the small molecule inhibitors PD173955 and imatinib (STI-571). Cancer Res 2002; 62:4236–4243.

13. Lombardo LJ, Lee FY, Chen P, et al. Discovery of N-(2-chloro-6-methyl- phenyl)-2-(6-(4-(2-hydroxyethyl)- piperazin-1-yl)-2-methylpyrimidin-4- ylamino)thiazole-5-carboxamide (BMS-354825), a dual Src/Abl kinase inhibitor with potent antitumor activity in preclinical assays. J Med Chem 2004; 47:6658–6661.

14. Lee F, Lombardo, L, Camuso, A, et al. BMS-354825 potently inhibits multiple selected oncogenic tyrosine kinases and possesses broad spectrum anti-tumor activities in vitro and in vivo. Proc Am Assoc Cancer Res 2005; 46:159(abstr 675).

15. Shah NP, Tran C, Lee FY, Chen P, Norris D, Sawyers CL. Overriding imatinib resistance with a novel ABL kinase inhibitor. Science 2004; 305:399–401.

16. O'Hare T, Walters DK, Stoffregen EP, et al. In vitro activity of Bcr-Abl inhibitors AMN107 and BMS-354825 against clinically relevant imatinib-resistant Abl kinase domain mutants. Cancer Res 2005; 65:4500–4505.

17. Burgess MR, Skaggs BJ, Shah NP, Lee FY, Sawyers CL. Comparative analysis of two clinically active *BCR-ABL* kinase inhibitors reveals the role of conformation-specific binding in resistance. Proc Natl Acad Sci USA 2005; 102:3395–3400.

18. Bradeen HA, Eide CA, O'Hare T, et al. Comparison of imatinib, dasatinib (BMS-354825), and nilotinib (AMN107) in an n-ethyl-n-nitrosourea (ENU)-based mutagenesis screen: high efficacy of drug combinations. Blood 2006; 108:2332–2338.

19. Hughes TP, Kaeda J, Branford S, et al. Frequency of major molecular responses to imatinib or interferon alfa plus cytarabine in newly diagnosed chronic myeloid leukemia. N Engl J Med 2003; 349:1423–1432.

20. Bhatia R, Holtz M, Niu N, et al. Persistence of malignant hematopoietic progenitors in chronic myelogenous leukemia patients in complete cytogenetic remission following imatinib mesylate treatment. Blood 2003; 101:4701–4707.

21. Graham S, Jorgensen HG, Allan E, et al. Primitive, quiescent, Philadelphia-positive stem cells from patients with chronic myeloid leukemia are insensitive to STI571 in vitro. Blood 2002; 99:319–325.

22. Holtz MS, Slovak ML, Zhang F, Sawyers CL, Forman SJ, Bhatia R. Imatinib mesylate (STI571) inhibits growth of primitive malignant progenitors in chronic myelogenous leukemia through reversal of abnormally increased proliferation. Blood 2002; 99:3792–3800.

23. Copland M, Hamilton A, Elrick LJ, et al. Dasatinib (BMS-354825) targets an earlier progenitor population than imatinib in primary CML, but does not eliminate the quiescent fraction. Blood 2006; 107:4532–4539.

24. Chu S, Xu H, Shah NP, et al. Detection of *BCR-ABL* kinase mutations in CD34+ cells from chronic myelogenous leukemia patients in complete cytogenetic remission on imatinib mesylate treatment. Blood 2005; 105:2093–2098.

25. Lee F, Wen ML, Camuso A, et al. Quiescent chronic myelogenous leukemia (CML) cells are resistant to *BCR-ABL* inhibitors but preferentially sensitive to BMS-214662, a farnesyltransferase inhibitor (FTI) with unique quiescent-cell selective cytotoxicity. Blood 2005; 106:(abstr 1993).

26. Gao H, Lee BN, Talpaz M, et al. Imatinib mesylate suppresses cytokine synthesis by activated CD4 T cells of patients with chronic myelogenous leukemia. Leukemia 2005; 19:1905–1911.

27. Gao H, Talpaz M, Lee N, et al. BMS-354825 induced complete hematologic remission in chronic phase CML patients without affecting T-cell cytokine production. J Clin Oncol 2005; 23:589s(abstr 6619).

28. Talpaz M, Kantarjian HM, Paquette R, et al. A phase I study of BMS-354825 in patients with imatinib-resistant and intolerant chronic phase chronic myeloid leukemia (CML): Results from CA180002. Proc Am Soc Clin Oncol 2005; 23:564s(abstr 6519).

29. Talpaz M, Shah NP, Kantarjian H, et al. Dasatinib in imatinib-resistant Philadelphia chromosome-positive leukemias. N Engl J Med 2006; 354:2531–2541.

30. Hochhaus A, Kantarjian H, Baccarini M, et al. Dasatinib efficacy and safety in patients with chronic phase CML resistant or intolerant to imatinib: Results of the CA180013 'START-C' phase II study. Proc Am Soc Clin Oncol 2006; 24:(abstr 6508).
31. Talpaz M, Apperley JF, Kim DW, et al. Dasatinib phase II study in patients with accelerated phase chronic myeloid leukemia (CML) who are resistant or intolerant to imatinib: results of the CA180005 'START-A' study. Proc Am Soc Clin Oncol 2006; 24:(abstr 6526).
32. Cortes J, Kim DW, Rosti G, et al. Dasatinib (D) in patients (pts) with chronic myelogenous leukemia (CML) in myeloid blast crisis (MBC) who are imatinib-resistant (IM-R) or IM-intolerant (IM-I): Results of the CA180006 'START-B' study. Proc Am Soc Clin Oncol 2006; 24:(abstr 6529).
33. Coutre S, Martinelli G, Dombret H, et al. Dasatanib (D) in patients (pts) with chronic myelogenous leukemia (CML) in lymphoid blast crisis (LB-CML) or Philadelphia-chromosome positive acute lymphoblastic leukemia (Ph + ALL) who are imatinib (IM)-resistant (IM-R) or intolerant (IM-I): The CA180015 'START-L' study. Proc Am Soc Clin Oncol 2006; 24:(abstr 6528).
34. Shah N, Rousselot P, Pasquini R, et al. Dasatinib (D) vs high dose imatinib (IM) in patients (pts) with chronic phase chronic myeloid leukemia (CP-CML) resistant to imatinib. Results of CA180017 START-R randomized trial. Proc Am Soc Clin Oncol 2006; 24:(abstr 6507).
35. Branford S, Hughes T, Nicoll J, et al. Major molecular responses to dasatinib (BMS-354825) are observed in imatinib-resistant late stage chronic and advanced CML patients: impact and fate of imatinib-resistant clones in dasatinib-treated patients. Blood 2005; 106:(abstr 437).
36. Quintas-Cardama A, Kantarjian H, Jones D, et al. Dynamics of molecular response to dasatinib (BMS-354825) in patients (pts) with chronic myelogenous leukemia (CML) resistant or intolerant to imatinib. Proc Am Soc Clin Oncol 2006; 24:(abstr 6525).

6 Nilotinib (AMN107) for the Treatment of Chronic Myelogenous Leukemia

Elias Jabbour, Francis Giles, Jorge Cortes, Susan O'Brien, and Hagop Kantarjian
Department of Leukemia, University of Texas M.D. Anderson Cancer Center, Houston, Texas, U.S.A.

INTRODUCTION

Chronic myelogenous leukemia (CML) is characterized by a balanced translocation, involving a fusion of the Abelson oncogene (ABL) from chromosome 9q34 with the breakpoint cluster region (BCR) on chromosome 22q11.2, t(9;22)(q34;q11.2), the Philadelphia chromosome (Ph). The molecular consequence of this translocation is the generation of a *BCR-ABL* fusion oncogene, which in turn translates into a Bcr-Abl oncoprotein. This most frequently has a molecular weight of 210 kD ($p210^{Bcr/Abl}$) and has increased tyrosine kinase activity, which is essential to its transforming capability (1,2). Imatinib mesylate is a potent and selective tyrosine kinase inhibitor that has become a standard therapy for patients with CML in all stages of the disease (2). A complete cytogenetic response (CCyR) can be achieved in 50% to 60% of patients treated in the chronic phase (CP) after failure of interferon-alpha (IFN-α) (3,4) and in over 80% of those receiving imatinib as first line therapy (5,6). Responses are durable in most patients treated in early CP, particularly among those who achieve major molecular responses (MMRs) (e.g., >3-log reduction in transcript levels) (7,8).

Despite the excellent results with imatinib in CML, resistance to this agent does occur in some cases at an annual rate of approximately 4% in newly diagnosed CML, but more often in advanced disease (9). Resistance may arise in several different ways, including *BCR-ABL*–dependent and *BCR-ABL*–independent mechanisms. The *BCR-ABL* kinase domain point mutations are often associated with imatinib resistance. These mutations impair imatinib activity, for example, by interfering with an imatinib-binding site or by stabilizing a conformation of Bcr-Abl with reduced affinity to imatinib (10,11). The Bcr-Abl kinase domain mutations vary in the extent to which they block imatinib binding and induce resistance to this drug (12,13).

Several approaches have been investigated to overcome resistance to imatinib, including the development of new, more potent tyrosine kinase inhibitors (14). Examples of such inhibitors under investigation include nilotinib (AMN107) (15), dasatinib (BMS-354825) (16), SKI-606 (17), INNO-406 (18), and AZD0530 (19). This chapter reviews the currently available data with nilotinib, including preclinical findings, pharmacokinetic data, results from phase I and phase II trials, possible indications beyond CML, and potential for use in combination therapy.

NILOTINIB

Nilotinib was developed using a rational design strategy based on the premise that Bcr-Abl inhibitors are more potent and selective than imatinib could be developed by making modest changes in this molecule (15). An analysis of the structure of imatinib and that of the Abl kinase domain indicated that changes to the structure's domain that binds deep into the adenosine triphosphate (ATP)-binding pocket would be likely to decrease its efficacy, but that modification of the methylpiperazinyl group of imatinib that lies along a partially hydrophobic group on the surface of Abl kinase might improve binding characteristics. Substitutions in this ring system resulted in the discovery of nilotinib, which is structurally similar to imatinib (Fig. 1) (20).

In Vitro Studies

Results from in vitro studies have demonstrated that nilotinib is more potent than imatinib in inhibiting Bcr-Abl tyrosine kinase activity in cell lines and that it is at least 10- to 30-fold more potent than imatinib in inhibiting proliferation of Bcr–Abl-expressing cells. Inhibition of cell growth by nilotinib was associated with induction of apoptosis, but it did not decrease the formation of normal human myeloid and erythroid progenitor cells at concentrations ≤ 100 μm (15).

Nilotinib effectively inhibited proliferation of Ba/F3 cells stably expressing point mutations (E255V, F317L, M351T, F486S, G250E, M244V, L248R, Q252H, Y253H, E255K, E279K, E282D, V289S, and L384M) associated with imatinib resistance in patients (Fig. 2). However, the T315I mutant remained resistant to nilotinib at concentrations <10 μM (15,21). Nilotinib also potently inhibited tyrosine autophosphorylation of the E255K, E255V, F317L, M351T, and F486S Bcr–Abl mutants, and these effects were not associated with decreases in Abl or Bcr–Abl protein levels. Overall, these results supported the conclusion that many imatinib-resistant Bcr–Abl mutants were relatively or absolutely more sensitive to nilotinib (22).

Nilotinib also inhibits, to a lesser extent, Pdgfrα and Pdgfrβ, as well as Kit dependent cell proliferation. In contrast, imatinib has more potency against Pdgfr and Kit than against Abl. Nilotinib has no significant activity against other kinases evaluated at concentrations <3000 nM (20).

Studies investigating the induction of mutants after exposure to imatinib under conditions that favor mutagenesis using a cell-based screen indicated that

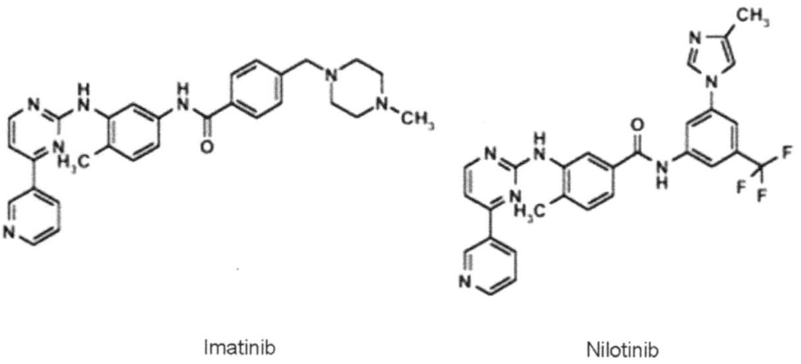

Imatinib   Nilotinib

FIGURE 1   Structural formulas for imatinib and nilotinib. *Source*: Adapted from Ref. 11.

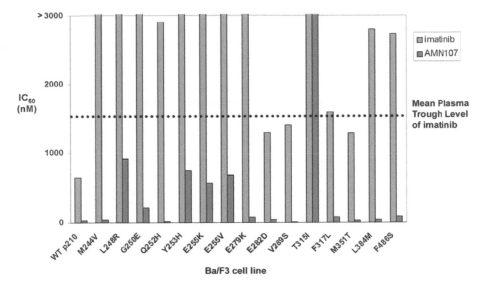

FIGURE 2 Comparison of imatinib and nilotinib IC_{50} values for blocking proliferation of Ba/F3 cells expressing wild-type Bcr-Abl or kinase domain mutated Bcr-Abl. *Note*: Solid gray bars indicate imatinib IC_{50} values, and solid red bars indicate nilotinib (AMN107) IC_{50} values. The dotted black line indicates the mean trough plasma level of imatinib reported in patients 24 hours following treatment with a once-daily dose of 400 mg. *Source*: Adapted from Ref. 31.

resistance to nilotinib was associated with a limited spectrum of Bcr-Abl kinase mutations, mostly affecting the P-loop and T315I. With the exception of T315I, all of the mutations identified in one study were effectively suppressed when the nilotinib concentration was increased to 2000 nM, which is within the trough-peak range for plasma levels (1.7–3.6 µM) measured in patients treated with nilotinib 400 mg twice daily. These results support the view that the clinical use of nilotinib has relatively low potential to result in significant resistance development by Bcr-Abl–expressing cells (23).

Additive or synergistic activity has been reported following the coadministration of imatinib and nilotinib in a panel of wild type and imatinib-resistant Bcr-Abl–expressing cell lines (24). This additive activity was confirmed in vivo in mice harboring 32D.p210 cells. Mice treated with both agents were observed to have a lower tumor burden than mice treated with either agent alone (24).

In Vivo Studies

The efficacy of nilotinib has been documented in in vivo models of CML, such as mice with Bcr-Abl–positive leukemias, both imatinib-sensitive and resistant. In both of these models, treatment with nilotinib significantly decreased tumor burden and prolonged survival relative to vehicle (15).

Pharmacokinetics

Results from pharmacokinetic studies in Balb/c mice given single doses of nilotinib of 20 or 75 mg/kg in 10% NMP/90% PEG300 by gavage indicated that the drug was orally bioavailable and well absorbed. These studies also demonstrated that nilotinib achieved high concentrations in both the liver and bone marrow (15).

The pharmacokinetics of nilotinib have been evaluated in a phase I dose-escalation study, in which 119 patients with imatinib-resistant Ph+ CML or acute lymphoblastic leukemia (ALL) received nilotinib as single oral daily (QD) doses of 50, 100, 200, 400, 800, or 1200 mg, or twice daily (BID) doses of 400 or 600 mg (25). The median time to peak serum concentrations of nilotinib was three hours, and the mean peak concentration at steady state (achieved at day eight) in patients administered 400 mg BID was 3.6 μM. Nilotinib had an apparent half-life of 15 hours. There was a 2-3-fold increase in exposure to nilotinib between the first dose and steady state. Peak concentration and area under the serum concentration–time curve at steady state increased with dose from 50 to 400 mg and plateaued with doses greater than 400 mg. Nonlinearity with higher nilotinib doses is thought to result from the saturation of gastrointestinal absorption; dosing nilotinib at 400 mg BID resulted in steady-state exposure greater than that observed with a single daily 800 mg dose (25). On the basis of this data, BID dosing was selected for phase II studies of nilotinib.

Clinical Results
Efficacy
Phase I
The phase I study of nilotinib included 119 patients with imatinib-resistant or intolerant Ph+ CML or ALL who received nilotinib QD at doses of 50, 100, 200, 400, 800, or 1200 mg, or 400 or 600 mg BID (25). Patients in this trial received nilotinib daily unless unacceptable adverse events or disease progression occurred. Intrapatient dose escalation was permitted in patients with an inadequate response and no dose-limiting toxicities (DLTs).

Efficacy results for patients with CML are summarized in Table 1. Overall, 39% of 33 patients with blastic phase CML achieved a hematologic response (HR), and 27% achieved a cytogenetic response. Among 46 patients with

TABLE 1 Phase I Hematologic and Cytogenetic Responses to Nilotinib in Patients with Chronic Myeloid Leukemia

Results in CML transformation	Total/ active[a]	CHR	MR	RTC	Overall	CR	PR	Minor	Minimal	Major	Overall
	Number (%) of hematologic response					Number (%) of cytogenetic response					
Accelerated phase											
Hematologic disease	46	21	3	9	33 (72)	6	3	4	9	9 (20)	22 (48)
Clonal evolution only[b]	10/5	5	—	—	5 (100)	2	4	1	2	6 (60)	9 (90)
Total	56/51	26	3	9	38 (74)	8	7	5	11	15 (27)	31(55)
Blastic phase											
Myeloid	24	2	2	6	10 (42)	1	4	2	—	(21)	(29)
Lymphoid	9	—	1	2	3 (33)	1	—	—	1	(11)	(22)
Total	33	2	3	8	13 (39)	2	4	2	1	6 (18)	9 (27)

[a]Patients with hematologic manifestation of disease (i.e., not CHR).
[b]Patients whose only criteria for accelerated phase was clonal evolution.
Abbreviations: CHR, complete hematologic response; CML, chronic myelogenous leukemia; CR, cytogenetic response; MR, major response; PR, partial response.

accelerated phase CML, excluding those with clonal evolution, 72% achieved a HR, and 48% had a cytogenetic response, including a major cytogenetic response in 20%. Six of 10 patients with clonal evolution achieved a major cytogenetic response. Of 17 patients with CP CML, 92% of 12 patients with active disease achieved complete hematologic response (CHR), and cytogenetic response was noted in 53% (complete in 35%) (Table 1) (25).

Fifty-one Abl kinase domain mutations were observed in 37 (41%) of 91 patients who were assessed at baseline. Hematologic and cytogenetic responses were similar in patients with or without mutations and in patients with p-loop or other mutations. The two patients with a T315I mutation did not respond to nilotinib (25).

Phase II
An ongoing, open-label phase II trial is evaluating nilotinib 400 mg BID in CML postresistance to or intolerance of imatinib. Preliminary data for 81 patients with CP CML (65% imatinib-resistant and 35% imatinib-intolerant) treated for a median of 185 days indicated that major cytogenetic responses were observed in 46% (32% complete, 14% partial), minor cytogenetic responses in 11%, and minimal cytogenetic responses in 11%. CHRs were observed in 69% of 54 patients without CHR at baseline (26). In accelerated phase CML ($n = 25$), HR was achieved in 40% and CHR in 16%. Cytogenetic responses were noted in 14 patients (4 complete, 3 partial, 2 minor, and 5 minimal) (27). This trial also included 24 patients in blastic phase and 16 patients with Ph+ ALL (15 relapsed/refractory, 1 minimal residual disease). HRs were reported for 12.5% in blastic phase (1 CHR, 1 marrow response/no evidence of leukemia, and 1 return to CP). Seven of the patients in blast phase had cytogenetic responses (5 complete and 2 partial). Complete remission was reported in 31% of patients with ALL (4 relapsed/refractory and 1 MRD) (28). A summary of the nilotinib-induced cytogenetic response for each phase of CML in these phase II studies is shown in Figure 3.

Nilotinib is also being investigated in patients with newly diagnosed CML (29). Fourteen patients with a median age of 49 received nilotinib 400 mg BID. Major cytogenetic response was observed in all patients at three months (complete in 13 and partial in 1). At six months all the seven evaluable patients were in CCyR. The treatment was well tolerated (29).

Nilotinib is also being investigated in patients with other hematologic malignancies. Twenty-four patients with systemic mastocytosis have been enrolled in a phase II study. Overall, 17% responded (2 complete remission and 1 minor response) and eight had stable disease, based on serum tryptase, bone marrow mast cell counts, and improvement of clinical symptoms (30).

Safety
In the phase I trial of nilotinib the maximum tolerated dose (MTD), defined as the highest dose of AMN107 given for at least one cycle in which ≤33% experienced a DLT, was 600 mg BID (25).

Nilotinib was generally well tolerated. The most common hematologic adverse events across all nilotinib doses were thrombocytopenia (21%) and neutropenia (14%), mainly grade 3 or 4. The frequency of both appeared to increase with nilotinib dose (25). Rash and pruritus were the most common nonhematologic adverse events (20% and 15% of patients, respectively), but were almost all grade 1 or 2 (25). The most common laboratory abnormalities were elevations in bilirubin

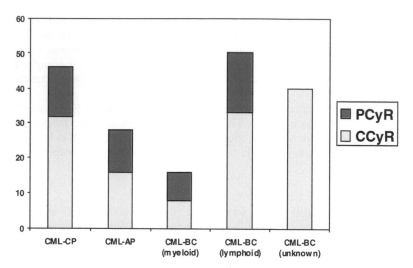

FIGURE 3 Phase II nilotinib response in imatinib-resistant/imatinib-intolerant chronic myelogenous leukemia (CML) patients. Phase II results showing percent of patients in each phase of CML. Chronic phase, accelerated phase, blast crisis (BC)-myeloid, BC-lymphoid, and BC-unknown) with complete and partial cytogenetic responses. *Abbreviations*: AP, accelerated phase; BC, blast crisis; CCyR, complete cytogenetic response; CML, chronic myelogenous leukemia; CP, chronic phase; PCyR, partial cytogenetic response.

(7% grade 1 or 2 and 7% grade 3 or 4), increased lipase (5% grade 3 or 4), and increased AST and/or ALT (1% grade 1 or 2 and 3% grade 3 or 4) (25). The frequency and grade of bilirubin elevations increased with nilotinib dose, but these rises were generally self-limiting and resolved with continued dosing of nilotinib (25). Analysis of ECGs indicated one instance of increased QTcF (5–15 msec). One patient had two treatment-related adverse cardiac events (grade 1 pericardial effusion and grade 2 atrial fibrillation) (25).

In the open-label phase II trial of nilotinib, adverse events that occurred in $\geq$10% of patients with CML included thrombocytopenia (32%), headache (29%), fatigue (29%), nausea (28%), pruritus (27%), rash (27%), anemia (26%), diarrhea (25%), neutropenia (21%), vomiting (20%), muscle spasms (20%), constipation and arthralgia (17% each), bone pain, myalgia, and peripheral edema (13% each), and abdominal pain and dyspepsia (12% each) (26–28).

Other Potential Indications for Nilotinib

Preclinical results suggest nilotinib may have clinical utility in other settings. Chronic myelmonocytic leukemia is associated with rearrangements of Pdgfrβ (31). Hyperesosinophilic syndrome is related to the FIP1L1–PDGFRα gene fusion (32). Some solid tumors, such as gastrointestinal solid tumors (GISTs), are associated with constitutive activation of Kit receptor tyrosine kinase (33). Recent results from Stover et al. have shown that nilotinib inhibits proliferation of Ba/F3 cells transformed by both TEL–PDGFRβ and FIP1L1–PDGFα with IC$_{50}$s <25 nM. Nilotinib also effectively treated myeloproliferative disease induced by TEL–PDGFRβ and FIP1L1–PDGFRα in an in vivo bone marrow transplant assay. In this model, nilotinib increased survival and disease latency and decreased disease severity as assessed by histopathology and flow cytometry (34). Nilotinib has also been demonstrated to inhibit proliferation of Ba/F3 cells transformed by a Kit (D814V) resistant to imatinib and known to be involved in systemic mast cell disease (35). Gleixner et al. (36) have reported similar results and also showed that nilotinib inhibited the proliferation of HMC-1 cells. These results suggest that nilotinib may be effective in the treatment of patients with chronic myelomonocytic leukemia, hypereosinophilic syndrome, systemic mastocytosis, or GIST. A phase I clinical trial of nilotinib in GIST is underway.

Use of Nilotinib in Combination Therapy

One ongoing clinical trial is evaluating the effectiveness of combination therapy with nilotinib plus imatinib in patients with GIST. A phase I dose escalation study of nilotinib in combination with imatinib in patients with CML in CP following a sub-optimal response to imatinib is ongoing.

CONCLUSIONS

Imatinib targets the tyrosine kinase activity of Bcr-Abl and is a breakthrough therapy that has dramatically altered the treatment of CML. Decreased efficacy of imatinib is often due to the emergence of clones expressing mutant forms of Bcr–Abl with reduced sensitivity to imatinib. The clinical importance of imatinib resistance and increased understanding of the structure of Abl and the molecular basis for resistance have resulted in the development of new agents active against Bcr–Abl mutants. Results from phase I and II clinical trials have demonstrated that nilotinib was effective and safe in patients with imatinib-resistant CML. Nilotinib may also be useful in the treatment of other conditions, such as chronic myelmonocytic leukemia, hypereosinophilic syndrome, systemic mastocytosis, or GIST.

REFERENCES

1. Faderl S, Talpaz M, Estrov Z, O'Brien S, Kurzrock R, Kantarjian HM. The biology of chronic myeloid leukemia. New Engl J Med 1999; 341:164–172.
2. Goldman JM, Melo JV. Chronic myeloid leukemia—advances in biology and new approaches to treatment. N Engl J Med 2003; 349:1451–1464.
3. Kantarjian HM, Cortes JE, O'Brien S, et al. Long-term survival benefit and improved complete cytogenetic and molecular response rates with imatinib mesylate in Philadelphia chromosome-positive chronic-phase chronic myeloid leukemia after failure of interferon-{alpha}. Blood 2004; 104:1979–1988.
4. Kantarjian H, Sawyers C, Hochhaus A, et al. Hematologic and cytogenetic responses to imatinib mesylate in chronic myelogenous leukemia. N Engl J Med 2002; 346:645–652.
5. O'Brien SG, Guilhot F, Larson RA, et al. Imatinib compared with interferon and low-dose cytarabine for newly diagnosed chronic-phase chronic myeloid leukemia. N Engl J Med 2003; 348:994–1004.
6. Kantarjian H, Talpaz M, O'Brien S, et al. High-dose imatinib mesylate therapy in newly diagnosed Philadelphia chromosome-positive chronic phase chronic myeloid leukemia. Blood 2004; 103:2873–2878.
7. Cortes J, Talpaz M, O'Brien S, et al. Molecular responses in patients with chronic myelogenous leukemia in chronic phase treated with imatinib mesylate. Clin Cancer Res 2005; 11:3425–3432.
8. Hughes TP, Kaeda J, Branford S, et al. Frequency of major molecular responses to imatinib or interferon alfa plus cytarabine in newly diagnosed chronic myeloid leukemia. N Engl J Med 2003; 349:1423–1432.

9. Manley PW, Cowan-Jacob SW, Mestan J. Advances in the structural biology, design and clinical development of Bcr-Abl kinase inhibitors for the treatment of chronic myeloid leukaemia. Biochim Biophys Acta 2005; 1754:3–13.
10. Hochhaus A, La Rosee P. Imatinib therapy in chronic myelogenous leukemia: strategies to avoid and overcome resistance. Leukemia 2004; 18:1–11.
11. Cowan-Jacob SW, Guez V, Griffin JD, et al. Bcr-Abl Kinase Mutations and Drug Resistance to Imatinib (STI571) in Chronic Myelogenous Leukemia. Mini Rev Med Chem 2004; 4:285–299.
12. Nicolini FE, Corm S, Le QH, et al. Mutation status and clinical outcome of 89 imatinib mesylate-resistant chronic myelogenous leukemia patients: a retrospective analysis from the French intergroup of CML (Fi(varphi)-LMC GROUP). Leukemia. 2006; 20:1061–1066.
13. Corbin AS, Buchdunger E, Pascal F, Druker BJ. Analysis of the structural basis of specificity of inhibition of the Abl kinase by STI571. J Biol Chem 2002; 277:32,214–32,219.
14. Golemovic M, Verstovsek S, Giles F, et al. AMN107, a novel aminopyrimidine inhibitor of Bcr-Abl, has in vitro activity against imatinib-resistant chronic myeloid leukemia. Clin Cancer Res 2005; 11:4941–4947.
15. Weisberg E, Manley PW, Breitenstein W, et al. Characterization of AMN107, a selective inhibitor of native and mutant Bcr-Abl. Cancer Cell 2005; 7:129–141.
16. Talpaz M, Shah N, Kantarjian HM, et al. Dasatinib in imatinib-resistant Philadelphia chromosome-positive leukemias. N Engl J Med 2006; 354:2531–2541.
17. Grafone T, Mancini M, Ottaqviani E, et al. A novel 4-anilino-3- quinolinecarbonitile dual SRC and ABL kinase inhibitor (SKI-606) has in vitro pro-apoptotic activity on CML Ph blast cells resistant to imatinib. Available at: http://www.parthen-impact.com/cgi-bin/pco/6_05EHA/publich/index.cgi?unit + pub_search_results&doem_i…
18. Kimura S, Naito H, Segawa H, et al. NS-187, a potent and selective dual Bcr-Abl/Lyn tyrosine kinase inhibitor, is a novel agent for imatinib-resistant leukemia. Blood 2005; 106:3948–3954.
19. Lockton JA, Smethurst D, Macpherson M, et al. Phase 1 ascending single and multiple dose studies to assess the safety, tolerability and pharmacokinetics of AZD0530, a highly selective, dual-specific SRC-ABL inhibitor. 2005. ASCO Annual Meeting.
20. O'Hare T, Walters DK, Deininger MW, Druker BJ. AMN107: tightening the grip of imatinib. Cancer Cell 2005; 7:117–119.
21. O'Hare T, Walters DK, Stoffregen EP, et al. In vitro activity of Bcr-Abl inhibitors AMN107 and BMS-354825 against clinically relevant imatinib-resistant Abl kinase domain mutants. Cancer Res 2005; 65:4500–4505.
22. Weisberg E, Manley P, Mestan J, Cowan-Jacob S, Ray A, Griffin JD. AMN107 (nilotinib): A novel and selective inhibitor Bcr-Abl. Br J Cancer 2006; 7:129–141.
23. von Bubnoff N, Manley PW, Mestan J, Sanger J, Peschel C, Duyster J. Bcr-Abl resistance screening predicts a limited spectrum of point mutations to be associated with clinical resistance to the Abl kinase inhibitor nilotinib (AMN107). Blood 2006; 108:1328–1333.
24. Griffin JD, Weisberg EL. Simultaneous administration of AMN107 and imatinib in the treatment of imatinib-sensitive and imatinib-resistant chronic myeloid leukaemia. Blood 2005;106:205a (abstract # 694).
25. Kantarjian H, Giles F, Wunderle L, et al. Nilotinib in imatinib-resistant CML and Philadelphia chromosome-positive ALL. N Engl J Med 2006; 354:2542–2551.
26. Kantarjian H, Gattermann N, O'Brien SG, et al. A phase II study of AMN107 (nilotinib), a novel inhibitor of Bcr-Abl, administered to imatinib resistant and intolerant patients (pts) with chronic myelogenous leukemia (CML) in chronic Phase (CP). ASCO 2006. Abstract 6534.
27. Le Coutre P, Ottmann O, GAttermann N, et al. A phase II study of AMN107 (nilotinib) a novel inhibitor of Bcr-Abl, administered to imatinib-resistant or intolerant patients with chronic myelogenous leukemia (CML) in accelerated phase (AP). ASCO 2006. Abstract 6531.
28. Giles F, Larson R, le Coutre P, et al. A phase II study of AMN107 (Nilotinib), a novel inhibitor of Bcr-Abl, administered to imatinib-resistant or intolerant patients with

chronic myelogenous leukemia (CML) in blast crisis (BC) or relapsed/refractory Ph+ acute lymphoblastic leukemia (ALL). ASCO 2006. Abstract 6536.

29. Jabbour E, Giles F, Cortes J, et al. Preliminary activity of AMN107, a novel potent oral selective Bcr-Abl tyrosine kinase inhibitor, in newly diagnosed Philadelphia chromosome (Ph)-positive chronic phase chronic myelogenous leukaemia (CML-CP). ASCO 2006. Abstract 6591.

30. Schatz M, Verhoef G, Gatterman. A phase II study of AMN107 (nilotinib), a novel tyrosine kinase inhibitor, administered to patients with systemic mastocytosis (SM). ASCO 2006. Abstract 6588.

31. Apperley JF, Gardembas M, Melo JV, et al. Response to imatinib mesylate in patients with chronic myeloproliferative diseases with rearrangements of the platelet-derived growth factor receptor beta. N Engl J Med 2002; 347:481–487.

32. Cools J, DeAngelo DJ, Gotlib J, et al. A tyrosine kinase created by fusion of the PDGFRA and FIP1L1 genes as a therapeutic target of imatinib in idiopathic hypereosinophilic syndrome. N Engl J Med. 2003; 348:1201–1214.

33. Demetri GD, von Mehren M, Blanke CD, et al. Efficacy and safety of imatinib mesylate in advanced gastrointestinal stromal tumors. N Engl J Med 2002; 347:472–480.

34. Stover EH, Chen J, Lee BH, et al. The small molecule tyrosine kinase inhibitor AMN107 inhibits TEL-PDGFRβ and FIP1L1-PDGFRα in vitro and in vivo. Blood 2005; 106:3206–3213.

35. von Bubnoff N, Gorantla SH, Kancha RK, Lordick F, Peschel C, Duyster J. The systemic mastocytosis-specific activating cKit mutation D816V can be inhibited by the tyrosine kinase inhibitor AMN107. Leukemia 2005; 19:1670–1671.

36. Gleixner KV, Mayerhofer M, Aichberger KJ, et al. PKC412 inhibits in vitro growth of neoplastic human mast cells expressing the D816V-mutated variant of KIT: comparison with AMN107, imatinib, and cladribine (2CdA) and evaluation of cooperative drug effects. Blood 2006; 107:752–759.

7 Resistance to Imatinib

Justus Duyster and Nikolas von Bubnoff

Department of Internal Medicine III, Klinikum rechts der Isar, Technical University of Munich, Munich, Germany

The mechanisms of imatinib resistance were first studied in cell culture-based systems. Bcr-Abl positive leukemic cells cultured in suboptimal concentrations of imatinib for prolonged periods of time developed moderate imatinib resistance to concentrations of up to approximately 1 μM (1–3). Further investigations revealed molecular changes possibly underlying resistance in these cell lines. During the imatinib selection process, these cells acquired amplification of the *BCR-ABL* gene or overexpression of MDR-1, which codes for a multidrug-resistance membrane associated transporter protein (1–3). Clinical resistance to imatinib, primarily occurring in advanced-phase CML and Ph-positive ALL, stimulated intensive studies to elucidate the mechanisms underlying resistance to imatinib in the clinic. In 2001, it was shown that 3 of 11 imatinib-resistant patients with advanced CML or Ph-positive ALL displayed amplification of the *BCR-ABL* gene (4). Furthermore, in 6 of 9 imatinib resistant patients a mutation in the *BCR-ABL* kinase domain was discovered, which leads to an amino acid exchange at position 315 from threonine to isoleucine (4). This amino acid exchange interferes with imatinib binding (5) and results in significant resistance against the drug (IC50> 10 μM) (4). Subsequently, a large number of additional *BCR-ABL* mutations could be identified causing variable degrees of imatinib resistance (6–11). Furthermore, in a study of 36 imatinib-resistant patients, cytogenetic abnormalities in addition to the Philadelphia (Ph) chromosome were noted, indicating that clonal evolution in an imatinib-resistant leukemic clone had occurred (7). Mechanisms of imatinib resistance observed both in cell lines and in clinical samples are summarized in Figure 1.

DEFINITION OF IMATINIB RESISTANCE

Primary resistance describes the failure to obtain a sufficient response despite adequate imatinib treatment. Primary hematologic resistance can be assumed if a patient does not achieve any hematologic response after three months or no complete hematologic response after six month, despite sufficient imatinib treatment. A primary cytogenetic resistance can be defined as a lack of any cytogenetic response after six month of treatment or no complete cytogentic response after 18 month. Secondary or acquired refers to loss of a previously established hematologic or cytogenetic remission. In addition, a molecular resistance or suboptimal molecular response may be defined as a lack of a major molecular response after 18 month or loss of a major molecular response, which should be confirmed on two occasions, unless associated with loss of hematologic or cytogenetic remission. Achievement of a major molecular response is assessed by measuring the absolute amount of *BCR-ABL* transcripts by quantitative RQ-PCR. However, it is important to note that the absolute amount of *BCR-ABL* transcripts, which corresponds to a major

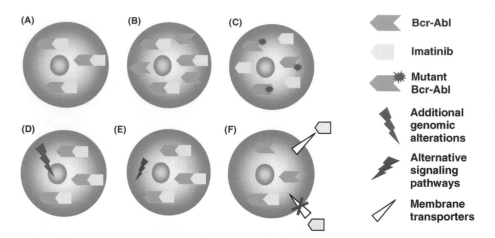

FIGURE 1   Mechanisms of resistance toward imatinib. (**A**) Imatinib is available within the cell at a sufficient quantity for inhibition of all Bcr-Abl-molecules. (**B**) Overexpression of Bcr-Abl allows the leukemic cell to maintain a baseline level of signaling that is sufficient for cell survival even in the presence of imatinib. (**C**) Specific mutations within the Abl kinase domain prevent binding of imatinib but still allow binding of ATP thus retaining Bcr-Abl kinase-active. (**D**) Secondary genetic alterations or (**E**) the activation of alternative signaling pathways contribute to the Bcr-Abl-independent growth and/or survival of the malignant clone. (**F**) Expression of membrane-bound transport proteins leads to deminished concentrations of inhibitor available within the cell by increased eflux or decreased influx.

molecular response, cannot consistently be determined, as yet, by different labora-tories in a comparable way. Attempts for an international harmonization of RQ-PCR results are an ongoing process (12,13).

INCIDENCE OF IMATINIB RESISTANCE

Primary hematologic resistance in early chronic phase CML is rare (<5 %). The fre-quency of secondary resistance in early chronic phase CML is also low. According to the international IRIS study group with a followup of 54 month, approximately 4% of patients per year in the imatinib arm had a progression event (14). Only 1% to 2% of the patients per year progressed to accelerated phase or blast phase CML (14). Similar percentages of patients per year lost a previously achieved hematologic or cytogenetic response. In this context it is important to note that there are no data to indicate that the number of resistant patients per year increases over time, in newly diagnosed patients with CML treated with imatinib. In other words, the compound does not seem to loose its activity with a followup of almost five years. However, assuming similar PFS kinetics in the future, the number of imatinib resistant patients will probably increase over time, albeit at a low rate.

The frequency of secondary imatinib resistance in patients who were initially treated with interferon in the IRIS trial but later on crossed over to imatinib is slightly higher at approximately 7% per year(14).

Compared to chronic phase, the results in advanced phases of CML are less impressive. In several large phase II studies, approximately one-third of patients with accelerated phase and two-third of patients with blastic phase CML showed primary hematologic resistance. Even if a hematologic or cytogenetic response was achieved, these responses were not frequently durable. Thus, after four years, 70% of AP patients and 90% of BP patients show a progression or secondary imatinib resistance (15–18). One needs to consider, though, that many of the patients treated in these trials had been pretreated extensively before starting imatinib, and the results may, therefore, be superior in newly diagnosed patients.

MECHANISMS OF IMATINIB RESISTANCE
BCR-ABL-Dependent Resistance
Mutations in the Kinase Domain of BCR-ABL

The first imatinib resistance mutation discovered leads to an exchange of threonine at position 315 to isoleucine (4). Interestingly, crystal structure analysis of the *ABL*-kinase domain published in 2000 had already predicted threonine 315 to be a critical position required for imatinib binding to *ABL* (5). Indeed, the T315I mutation leads to complete biochemical imatinib resistance, even at high imatinib concentrations, while the kinase activity is preserved (4). In recent times, more than 40 different imatinib-resistance mutations have been described. Mutations in the *BCR-ABL* kinase domain can be identified in 42% to 90% of cases with imatinib-resistant CML or Ph-positive ALL (4,6,9–11,19). All mutations identified in imatinib-resistant patients so far are located within the *BCR-ABL* kinase domain. They lead to structural changes so that imatinib is no longer able to displace ATP, thereby preserving kinase activity.

Imatinib resistance mutations can be divided into two distinct groups:

1. Imatinib-contact positions such as Y253, T315, and F317. This class of mutations affects amino acids, which are directly involved in binding of the drug. Mutations at these positions thus directly impede drug binding.
2. Mutations that destabilize the inactive conformation of *BCR-ABL*. These may include exchanges at positions located within the activation loop, such as H396 and M388, or mutations of SH2-contact positions, such as S348 or M351. This second class of mutations probably shifts the equilibrium toward the active state. Since imatinib binds only the inactive conformation of ABL with the activation loop in a closed conformation (5), access of imatinib to the ATP-binding site is impaired (10,11,20).

Mutations directly affecting imatinib binding typically lead to strong imatinib resistance. Examples are T315I and Y253H (4,11). In contrast, mutations, which stabilize the inactive conformation such as H396P, often lead only to moderate resistance (10,11,20). Thus, the type of mutation may affect therapeutic management in case of imatinib resistance. Increasing the dose of imatinib may be sufficient to block moderately resistant Bcr-Abl mutants. However, in the event of a strong imatinib-resistance mutation, increasing the dose will not achieve plasma concentrations that are sufficient to effectively block *BCR-ABL* kinase activity. Table 1 shows the degree of imatinib resistance for frequently observed mutations.

Another classification of resistance mutations is based on localization within the kinase domain:

1. Mutations in the activation loop (A-loop, magenta in Fig. 2)
2. Mutations in the ATP phosphate-binding loop (P-loop, pink in Fig. 2)
3. Mutations in the C-Helix (green in Fig. 2)

TABLE 1 Cellular IC50-Values of Frequently Observed Imatinib
Resistance Mutations

Mutation	Imatinib (μM)	Factor IC50 wt
Wild-type	0.4	—
P-loop		
M244V	2.3	5.8
L248V	1.5	3.8
G250E	3.9	7.5
Q252H	1.2	3
Y253H	>10	>25
Y253F	9	22.5
E255K	10	25
E255V	>10	>25
C-helix		
D276G	1.5	3.8
F311L	1.3	3.25
T315I	>10	>25
T315S	3.8	9.5
F317L	1.5	3.8
SH2-contact		
D325 N	1.5	3.8
S348L	0.7	1.4
M351T	4.9	12.25
M351I	1.6	4
E355G	0.4	1
F359C	1.2	3
F359V	1.2	3
A-loop		
L387F	1.1	2.8
H396P	2.5	6.25

IC50-values are based on studies performed in cell lines, which express
BCR-ABL mutations that were identified in patients with CML or Ph+ ALL and
resistance to imatinib (*Source*: From Refs. 4,10,11,59,75). Imatinib resistance
mutations in up to 50 per cent of the cases are located within the nucleotide-
binding loop (P-loop), with Y253 and E255 being most frequently affected. The
most abundant exchanges affecting single positions are T315I (20% of cases)
and M351T (15% of cases) (*Source*: From Refs. 21,84).

This classification does not allow in estimating the degree of resistance. As an example, the class of P-loop mutations includes moderately (G250A, Q252H, E255D) as well as highly (G250E, Y253H, E255V) imatinib-resistance mutations (10,21).

Meanwhile, mutations conferring clinical resistance to therapeutically used kinase inhibitors were also identified in several other target kinases in various malignant diseases. Imatinib resistance mutations were identified in FIP1L1-PDGFR alpha in patients with hypereosinophilic syndrome (23,24), and in cKit in patients with gastrointestinal stromal tumors (GIST) (25,26). In addition, a resistance mutation in the kinase domain of FLT3 in a patient with acute myeloid leukemia (AML) treated with the kinase inhibitor PKC412 has been described (27). Similarly, in patients with non small cell lung cancer (NSCL), treated with the kinase inhibitor gefitinib (Iressa), an exchange of threonine at position 790 to methionine in the epidermal growth factor receptor (EGFR) was described (28,29). This mutation, together with the imatinib-resistant mutations KIT/T670I and FIP1L1-PDGFRalpha/T674I, is homologous to position T315 in the ABL-kinase domain,

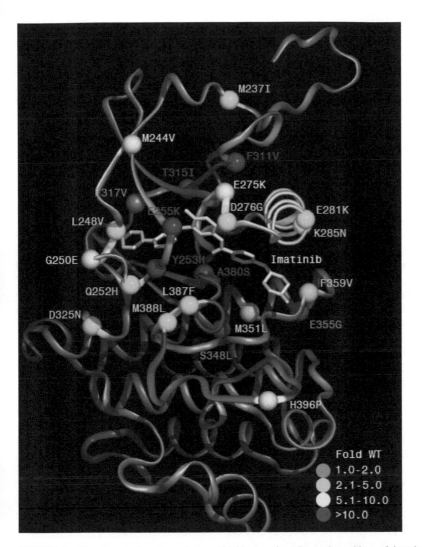

FIGURE 2 Functional domains of the Abl kinase domain and position of imatinib resistance mutations. Ribbon representation of the c-Abl kinase domain in complex with imatinib, with C-helix in light green, P-loop in pink, and A-loop in magenta, with the A-loop in an open conformation. Labels indicate the residue number of human c-Abl kinase type Ia. The colors of the spheres represent the degree of cellular resistance to imatinib expressed as fold cellular IC50 of wild-type Bcr-Abl in Ba/F3 cells. *Source*: Adapted from Ref. 21.

confirming the critical role of this residue for the binding of ATP-competitive kinase inhibitors. Thus, mutations in kinase domains appear to be a general mechanism of resistance against tyrosine kinase inhibitors.

BCR-ABL *Gene Amplification and Protein Overexpression*
BCR-ABL gene amplification and protein overexpression as causes of imatinib resistance were both identified in vitro (1–3) as well as in CML patient samples

(4,29). Amplification of a kinase inhibitor target could also be demonstrated for KIT in imatinib-resistant GIST patients (30). Amplification of the target gene results in a shift of the inhibitor/target ratio toward a surplus of the target protein. Consequently, the amount of inhibitor available within the cell is not sufficient to effectively block all target protein molecules. In the case of CML, *BCR-ABL* overexpression allows for residual kinase activity even in the presence of imatinib, which enables the leukemic clone to survive.

Phamacokinetic- and Drug Transport-Issues

Alterations in the distribution of imatinib and its delivery to target cells can result in suboptimal drug concentrations within leukemic cells and thereby may give rise to resistant disease. The intracellular concentration of imatinib is determined by membrane-bound, active import and export pumps, and by its binding to plasma proteins. It was shown that imatinib is bound to plasma proteins, such as α-1-acid-glycoprotein (α-1-GP) (31). It has been proposed that increased plasma α-1-GP levels might reduce the plasma concentration of free unbound imatinib that is available for inhibition of *BCR-ABL* (31). Indeed, the tumor burden in a mouse model (32) and the CML disease stage in patients (33) correlated with plasma α-1-GP levels and elevated α-1-GP levels prior to treatment led to a less rapid response to imatinib in CML patients (33). However, elevated α-1-GP plasma levels in patients were reversible in the course of treatment (33), and α-1-GP did not alter the efficacy of the drug in vitro (33,34). Therefore, it is currently unclear whether plasma proteins such as α-1-GP contribute to imatinib resistance or not.

Imatinib is a substrate of the multi drug resistance-associated membrane transporter MDR-1 and thus can be actively pumped out of the cell (35,36). Overexpression of MDR-1 was found in imatinib-resistant cell lines, and by inhibition of MDR-1 imatinib resistance was partially reverted (2). Increased expression of MDR-1 was also demonstrated on progenitor cells of patients with CML in myeloid blast crisis when compared to healthy controls, although the level of expression did not predict response to imatinib. In contrast, low levels of MRP-1, another drug transporter, correlated with response to treatment (37). Recently, a membrane transporter was identified (*human organic cation transporter-1*; hOCT-1), which may be involved in the active transport of imatinib into the cell (import) (38). A small study demonstrated a correlation of hOCT-1 expression and response to imatinib (39). Larger studies are required to substantiate the impact of hOCT-1 expression for imatinib activity.

On the whole, drug transport mechanisms may be of potential importance for the survival of CML cells in the presence of imatinib. However, clinical evidence that pharmacokinetic mechanisms play an important role for imatinib resistance is still inconclusive, since no single critical mechanism has been identified. However, it is conceivable that pharmacokinetic mechanisms may be important for a cell in the course of acquiring secondary resistance due to mutations or secondary genetic alterations in the presence of imatinib.

Compliance

Patient compliance is an issue with any continuously administered drug as adherence to medications usually declines with time. A survey by Novartis estimated that up to one-third of drug doses might have been actually missed. It is thought that poor compliance in the case of imatinib may lead to secondary resistance, because suboptimal drug concentrations may facilitate the selection of resistant leukemia clones. Patients with a good response particularly need to be reminded that it is important to continue the treatment, because discontinuation can lead to disease recurrence or development of resistance. Evidently, it is crucial to rule out noncompliance before changing therapy for suspected acquired resistance, particularly if less well-tolerated or risky alternative strategies are considered.

BCR-ABL-Independent Mechanisms of Resistance
Secondary Genetic Alterations, Alternative Pathways

In a small subset of imatinib resistant patients, it can be shown that the drug still effectively blocks *BCR-ABL* kinase activity. This indicates that the leukemia has become at least partially *BCR-ABL* independent as a result of secondary genetic events. Clonal cytogenetic evolution is frequently associated with imatinib resistance (7,40,41) and has been demonstrated to be an independent poor prognostic factor for survival in CML (42). However, the molecular mechanisms by which specific chromosomal alterations lead to resistance are not understood. Two frequently described cytogenetic abnormalities are isochromosome 17, leading to inactivation of p53 (43,44), and trisomy 8, resulting in amplification and overexpression of MYC (45). Both events may contribute to disease progression and imatinib resistance (45–47). In one imatinib-resistant CML patient, an inversion of chromosome 11 [inv(11)(p15q22)] led to the expression of a NUP98/DDX10 fusion protein (48). Interestingly, NUP98/DDX10 is also associated with AML and myelodysplastic syndromes and, thus, may play a functional important role for disease progression and imatinib resistance (49).

The finding of LYN kinase overexpression in bone-marrow samples derived from imatinib resistant CML patients suggested that activation of SRC family kinases may bypass the dependence of the leukemic cell on active *BCR-ABL,* and thus may contribute to imatinib resistance (50). Since some of these data are based on cell lines, established from patients, it is not entirely clear how relevant SRC kinase activation is for the imatinib resistance of primary cells. Regardless of this, it is evident that *BCR-ABL* kinase domain mutations and overexpression fail to explain acquired and, all the more, primary resistance in a significant number of patients.

Prevention of Resistance

Since nearly all patients with chronic phase CML have persistent disease as indicated by the presence of *BCR-ABL* transcripts (51), it is critical to maintain sufficient *BCR-ABL* kinase inhibition in order to reduce the risk of disease progression or development of resistant disease. Moreover, the IRIS trial has shown that newly diagnosed CML chronic phase patients who received imatinib as their initial therapy had superior cytogenetic response and overall survival than patients who first received interferon and later on crossed over to imatinib (14). Therefore, it is recommended to initiate treatment immediately after diagnosis with 400 mg per day in chronic phases and 600 mg in advanced phases. It is important to avoid unnecessary dose reductions or interruptions. Whenever possible, imatinib side effects should be treated without dose reduction. If a dose reduction is inevitable, doses lower than 300 mg per day should be avoided. Below a daily dose of 300 mg, imatinib plasma levels are not sufficient to suppress *BCR-ABL* kinase activity (52), which in turn may lead to the selection of resistant subclones.

Overriding Imatinib Resistance
Increasing the Imatinib Dose
In case of a suboptimal response to imatinib, the dose may be increased (53,54). Treatment guidelines have been proposed to identify patients who may benefit from a dose escalation (12,55). When resistance to imatinib emerges, the BCR-ABL kinase domain should be sequenced. If a mutation mediating moderate imatinib resistance is identified, increasing the dose to 600 or 800 mg is one therapeutic option. The degree of resistance for most mutations is known from in vitro studies, and the published IC50 values for different BCR-ABL mutations can be used as a guideline (Table 1). In the case of mutations other than P-loop or T315I, increasing the imatinib dose was reported to improve or stabilize the disease in a proportion of patients (56). This benefit was of shorter duration in P-loop mutant cases, and patients expressing T315I did not benefit from increasing the dose of imatinib.

Alternative ABL Inhibitors
Recently, additional compounds have been developed that inhibit BCR-ABL more potently than imatinib, and display activity against the majority of known imatinib resistance mutants. Results of ongoing clinical studies indicate that these theoretical advantages, indeed, might translate into clinical activity. However, whether the use of novel agents like AMN107 (nilotinib) or BMS-354825 (dasatinib) also generate superior response rates and long-term results in early chronic phase CML, remains to be shown. During the past years, several strategies have been employed to identify drugs with improved antileukemic activity that could be used in CML and Ph+ ALL. Agents may be subdivided into several subcategories:

1. Compounds that are similar to imatinib binding BCR-ABL in an inactive conformation but achieving a higher potency by an optimized fit to the ATP-binding site. An example is nilotinib (AMN107), which has been demonstrated to inhibit many of the known imatinib-resistant mutations, except T315I (57–59). Nilotinib has entered phase 2 clinical trials, and phase 1 data show promising activity in imatinib resistant, intolerant CML, or Ph + ALL (60).
2. Compounds that bind to both the inactive and active conformation irrespective of the A-loop conformation (closed versus open). Dasatinib (BMS-354825, Sprycel^{TM}) constitutes an example of this class (61,62). Dasatinib, similar to nilotinib, inhibits many of the known imatinib-resistant forms of BCR-ABL, except T315I (63). Dasatinib displayed significant activity in phase 1 studies of CML and Ph+ ALL (64) and is currently being evaluated in phase 2 clinical studies. Dasatinib was recently approved by the FDA for the treatment of adults in all phases of CML with resistance or intolerance to prior therapy, including imatinib. Pyrido-pyrimidines analogues also belong to this class of compounds (65–69). However, there are currently no plans for clinical evaluation of these compounds.
3. Dual SRC/ABL kinase inhibitors, in addition to BCR-ABL, inhibit other target kinases that may be important for the survival of the malignant clone. Examples for this group of compounds are dasatinib (BMS-354825, Sprycel^{TM}, see earlier), pyrido-pyrimidines analogues (mentioned earlier), SKI-606 (70), which recently entered phase 1 clinical evaluation, and INNO-406 [former NS-187 (72)].
4. Compounds that do not act as ATP-competitors but are thought to act as allosteric inhibitors binding to sites different from the ATP-binding pocket.

An example is ON012380, which is thought to act as a substrate competitor (73). The compound might be operational against imatinib-resistant *BCR-ABL* mutations, including T315I, and is currently in preclinical development. The allosteric inhibitor GNF-2 also belongs to this category (74). Inhibition by this agent may be attained by binding to the myristate binding moiety, thereby, capturing the kinase in an inactive state. The compound displayed activity against some of the tested imatinib resistant mutant forms of *BCR-ABL* (74).

5. Agents that show activity against the T315I mutation. A high throughput screen identified the aurora-kinase inhibitor VX-680 (MK-0457) to inhibit *BCR-ABL* T315I (75,21). A phase 1 clinical study with this compound has been launched. Also the non-ATP-competitive inhibitor ON012380 described earlier was reported to suppress T315I (72).

Thus, a large number of alternative *BCR-ABL* kinase inhibitors with divergent mode of actions are currently in preclinical or clinical development. Phase 1 clinical studies already demonstrated that AMN107 (nilotinib) and BMS-354825 (dasatinib) display activity in imatinib resistant cases, with and without the presence of *BCR-ABL* mutations (59,62). A large number of in vitro studies showed that novel ABL-kinase inhibitors like PD166326 (65,68), PD180970 (66), AMN107 (nilotinib) (57), BMS354825 (dasatinib) (64), AP23464 (71), SK1-606 (70) NS-187 (currently INNO-406) (72), ON012380 (73), or VX-680 (75) are capable of suppressing known imatinib resistant mutant forms of *BCR-ABL*. This well agrees with comparative crystal structure analysis indicating that different compounds display distinct binding modes to the ABL kinase domain (59,61,62,67), suggesting that different scaffolds may display specific patterns of resistance mutations. Knowing these scaffold specific resistance patterns may allow tailoring treatment strategies with respect to drug combinations in the future, which might reduce the frequency of resistance. In vitro screening strategies for imatinib resistance mutations in *BCR-ABL* have been developed that revealed specific mutation profiles for various ABL kinase inhibitors (22,76–80). These studies indicated that alternative ABL kinase inhibitors in comparison to imatinib indeed might display a limited, albeit overlapping, pattern of mutations. Indeed, the use of drug combinations narrowed the spectrum of *BCR-ABL* mutations emerging in vitro (77–79). Thus, specific mutation profiles for ABL kinase inhibitors can be generated in vitro, and this information may be translated into treatment strategies in the future that hopefully will minimize the emergence of drug resistance.

However, as mentioned earlier, it is important to keep in mind that most novel compounds do not overcome resistance to the T315I mutant. Therefore, patients with T315I should not be treated within these trials, unless studies are available where drug candidates with documented T315I activity are examined. One compound with reported T315I activity that has entered a phase 1 study is VX-680 (MK-0457) (Vertex Pharmaceuticals/Merck).

Allogenic Stem Cell Transplantation

Allogenic stem cell transplantation in the era of specific ABL kinase inhibitors is becoming increasingly infrequent and always constitutes an individual decision. Allogeneic transplant should be considered in case of imatinib resistant relapse preferentially after achieving a remission with an alternative ABL kinase inhibitor.

PERSISTENCE OF DISEASE

Imatinib is currently not considered a curative treatment. The majority of patients do not achieve PCR negativity (13). Imatinib discontinuation usually leads to disease recurrence even in the case of a good molecular response. The BCR-ABL-positive cell population that persists despite continuous imatinib treatment is not well defined. It is thought that residual leukemia cells reside in an early progenitor or stem-cell compartment, although a precise characterization of this compartment is lacking. It is known that CML patients harbor primitive BCR-ABL-positive progenitor cells that infrequently undergo cell division (81) and are thus referred to as quiescent cells. In vitro studies suggest that these quiescent cells do not depend on kinase active BCR-ABL for survival and therefore are resistant to imatinib (82,83). Additional events might be active in these persisting cells such as mutations, drug efflux pumps or constitutive activation of alternative survival signaling cascades, cooperating in the constitution of a resistant disease clone. Recently, it has been shown that BCR-ABL kinase domain mutations can be detected in progenitor cells derived from CML patients in complete cytogenetic remission on imatinib (84). Since persistent disease represents the point of origin for relapse and resistance, it will be crucial to characterize this cell population in more detail and to elucidate the mechanisms by which these immature cells evade eradication. These studies will be the prerequisite for the development of rational therapeutic strategies that may ultimately allow the cure of CML.

CONCLUSIONS

CML has become the paradigm for targeted cancer treatment. The introduction of imatinib has led to a dramatic improvement of prognosis in chronic phase patients when compared to conventional chemotherapy. The use of small molecule kinase inhibitors has been extended to other entities, and thereby redefined the management of cancer, in general. By virtue of their specific mode of action and the addiction of CML to BCR-ABL, resistance to therapeutic kinase inhibitors is based on a limited number of mechanisms that were elucidated by focusing on changes taking place at the target kinase itself. This scenario is completely different from conventional chemotherapy, where resistance is of multifactorial origin, and detection of resistance mechanisms generally does not have an immediate impact on further treatment. In contrast, understanding resistance in kinase inhibitor based therapies clearly affects subsequent treatment, since specific point mutations may prevent binding of a certain class of compounds, while a structurally different substances still can bind and do its job. When amplification of the BCR-ABL gene occurs, higher doses of a kinase inhibitor may overcome residual BCR-ABL activity. Therefore, detection of specific mechanisms of resistance in an individual patient certainly has an immediate impact on further treatment, and the determination of individual resistance profiles for different classes of BCR-ABL kinase inhibitors allows the design of sequential or combinatorial treatment strategies, thereby limiting the number of possible "escape" mutations. Once resistance to imatinib has occurred, sequencing of the BCR-ABL kinase may demonstrate a resistance mutation, and switching to an appropriate alternate compound may overcome a mutated disease clone.

   The finding of target kinase domain mutations giving rise to resistance toward kinase inhibitors has been reproduced in other examples of targeted cancer treatments. Examples are NSCL, where exchanges in the EGFR kinase domain can abrogate binding and inhibition of EGFR kinase inhibitors such as gefitinib, and mutations in KIT or FIP1L1-PDGFRalpha in imatinib resistant gastrointestinal stromal tumor (GIST), or chronic eosinophilic leukemia, respectively. Understanding molecular changes underlying resistance to therapeutically used kinase inhibitors will undoubtedly improve treatment strategies. Applying this knowledge to the individual patient requires cytogenetic and molecular monitoring, including mutational analysis.

REFERENCES

1. le Coutre P, Tassi E, Varella-Garcia M, et al., and Gambacorti-Passerini C. Induction of resistance to the Abelson inhibitor STI571 in human leukemic cells through gene amplification. Blood 2000; 95:1758–1766.
2. Mahon FX, Deininger MW, Schultheis B, et al. Selection and characterization of *BCR-ABL* positive cell lines with differential sensitivity to the tyrosine kinase inhibitor STI571: diverse mechanisms of resistance. Blood 2000; 96:1070–1079.
3. Weisberg E, Griffin JD. Mechanism of resistance to the ABL tyrosine kinase inhibitor STI571 in *BCR/ABL*-transformed hematopoietic cell lines. Blood 2000; 95:3498–3505.
4. Gorre ME, Mohammed M, Ellwood K, Hsu N, Paquette R, Rao PN, Sawyers CL. Clinical resistance to STI-571 cancer therapy caused by *BCR-ABL* gene mutation or amplification. Science 2001; 293:876–880.
5. Schindler T, Bornmann W, Pellicena P, Miller WT, Clarkson B, Kuriyan J. Structural mechanism for STI-571 inhibition of abelson tyrosine kinase. Science 2000; 289:1938–1942.
6. Branford S, Rudzki Z, Walsh S, et al. High frequency of point mutations clustered within the adenosine triphosphate-binding region of *BCR/ABL* in patients with chronic myeloid leukemia or Ph-positive acute lymphoblastic leukemia who develop imatinib (STI571) resistance. Blood 2002; 99:3472–3475.
7. Hochhaus A, Kreil S, Corbin AS, et al. Molecular and chromosomal mechanisms of resistance to imatinib (STI571) therapy. Leukemia 2002; 16:2190–2196.
8. Hofmann WK, Komor M, Wassmann B, et al. Presence of the *BCR-ABL* mutation Glu255Lys prior to STI571 (imatinib) treatment in patients with Ph+ acute lymphoblastic leukemia. Blood 2003; 102:659–661.
9. Roche-Lestienne C, Soenen-Cornu V, Grardel-Duflos N, et al. Several types of mutations of the Abl gene can be found in chronic myeloid leukemia patients resistant to STI571, and they can pre-exist to the onset of treatment. Blood 2002; 100:1014–1018.
10. Shah NP, Nicoll JM, Nagar B, et al. Multiple *BCR-ABL* kinase domain mutations confer polyclonal resistance to the tyrosine kinase inhibitor imatinib (STI571) in chronic phase and blast crisis chronic myeloid leukemia. Cancer Cell 2002; 2:117–125.
11. von Bubnoff N, Schneller F, Peschel C, Duyster J. *BCR-ABL* gene mutations in relation to clinical resistance of Philadelphia-chromosome-positive leukaemia to STI571: a prospective study. Lancet 2002; 359:487–491.
12. Baccarani M, Saglio G, Goldman J, et al. Evolving concepts in the management of chronic myeloid leukemia. Recommendations from an expert panel on behalf of the European Leukemianet. Blood 2006; 108:1809–1820.
13. Hughes T, Deininger M, Hochhaus, et al. Monitoring CML patients responding to treatment with tyrosine kinase inhibitors: review and recommendations for harmonizing current methodology for detecting *BCR-ABL* transcripts and kinase domain mutations and for expressing results. Blood 2006; 108:28–37.
14. Simonsson B. Beneficial effects of cytogenetic and molecular response on longterm outcome in patients with newly diagnosed chronic myeloid leukemia in chronic phase (CML-CP) treated with imatinib (IM): update from the IRIS study. The IRIS study group. Blood 2005; 106:52a.
15. Druker BJ, Sawyers CL, Kantarjian, et al. Activity of a specific inhibitor of the *BCR-ABL* tyrosine kinase in the blast crisis of chronic myeloid leukemia and acute

lymphoblastic leukemia with the Philadelphia chromosome. N Engl J Med 2001; 344:1038–1042.

16. Kantarjian HM, Cortes J, O'Brien S, et al. Imatinib mesylate (STI571) therapy for Philadelphia chromosome-positive chronic myelogenous leukemia in blast phase. Blood 2002; 99:3547–3553.

17. Kantarjian HM, O'Brien S, Cortes JE, et al. Treatment of philadelphia chromosome-positive, accelerated-phase chronic myelogenous leukemia with imatinib mesylate. Clin Cancer Res 2002; 8:2167–2176.

18. Ottmann OG, Druker BJ, Sawyers CL, et al. A phase 2 study of imatinib in patients with relapsed or refractory Philadelphia chromosome-positive acute lymphoid leukemias. Blood 2002; 100:1965–1971.

19. Hochhaus A, La Rosee P. Imatinib therapy in chronic myelogenous leukemia: strategies to avoid and overcome resistance. Leukemia 2004; 18:1321–1331.

20. Young MA, Shah NP, Chao LH, et al. Structure of the kinase domain of an imatinib-resistant Abl mutant in complex with the Aurora kinase inhibitor VX-680. Cancer Res 2006; 66:1007–1014.

21. von Bubnoff N, Veach DR, van der Kuip H, et al. A cell-based screen for resistance of Bcr-Abl-positive leukemia identifies the mutation pattern for PD166326, an alternative Abl kinase inhibitor. Blood 2005; 105:1652–1659.

22. Cools J, DeAngelo DJ, Gotlib J, et al. A tyrosine kinase created by fusion of the PDGFRA and FIP1L1 genes as a therapeutic target of imatinib in idiopathic hypereosinophilic syndrome. N Engl J Med 2003; 348:1201–1214.

23. von Bubnoff N, Sandherr M, Schlimok G, Andreesen R, Peschel C, Duyster J. Myeloid blast crisis evolving during imatinib treatment of an FIP1L1-PDGFR alpha-positive chronic myeloproliferative disease with prominent eosinophilia. Leukemia 2005; 19:286–287.

24. Chen LL, Trent JC, Wu EF, et al. A missense mutation in KIT kinase domain 1 correlates with imatinib resistance in gastrointestinal stromal tumors. Cancer Res 2004; 64:5913–5919.

25. Tamborini E, Bonadiman L, Greco A, et al. A new mutation in the KIT ATP pocket causes acquired resistance to imatinib in a gastrointestinal stromal tumor patient. Gastroenterology 2004; 127:294–299.

26. Heidel F, Breitenbuecher F, Kindler T, et al. Mechanisms of resistance to the FLT3-tyrosine kinase inhibitor PKC412 in patients with AML. Blood 2004; 104:133a.

27. Kobayashi S, Boggon TJ, Dayaram T, et al. EGFR mutation and resistance of non-small-cell lung cancer to gefitinib. N Engl J Med 2005; 352:786–792.

28. Shih JY, Gow CH, and Yang PC. EGFR mutation conferring primary resistance to gefitinib in non-small-cell lung cancer. N Engl J Med 2005; 353:207–208.

29. Hochhaus A. Cytogenetic and molecular mechanisms of resistance to imatinib. SeminHematol 2003; 40:69–79.

30. Debiec-Rychter M, Cools J, Dumez H, et al. Mechanisms of resistance to imatinib mesylate in gastrointestinal stromal tumors and activity of the PKC412 inhibitor against imatinib-resistant mutants. Gastroenterology 2005; 128:270–279.

31. Capdeville R, Buchdunger E, Zimmermann J, Matter A. Glivec (STI571, imatinib), a rationally developed, targeted anticancer drug. Nat Rev Drug Discov 2002; 1:493–502.

32. Gambacorti-Passerini C, Barni R, le Coutre P, et al. Role of alpha1 acid glycoprotein in the in vivo resistance of human BCR-ABL(+) leukemic cells to the abl inhibitor STI571. J Natl Cancer Inst 2000; 92:1641–1650.

33. le Coutre P, Kreuzer KA, Na IK, et al. Determination of alpha-1 acid glycoprotein in patients with Ph+ chronic myeloid leukemia during the first 13 weeks of therapy with STI571. Blood Cells Mol Dis 2002; 28:75–85.

34. Jorgensen HG, Elliott MA, Allan EK, Carr CE, Holyoake TL, Smith KD. Alpha1-acid glycoprotein expressed in the plasma of chronic myeloid leukemia patients does not mediate significant in vitro resistance to STI571. Blood 2002; 99:713–715.

35. Fromm MF. Importance of P-glycoprotein at blood-tissue barriers. Trends Pharmacol Sci 2004; 25:423–429.

36. Sparreboom A, Danesi R, Ando Y, Chan J, Figg WD. Pharmacogenomics of ABC trans-porters and its role in cancer chemotherapy. Drug Resist Updat 2003; 6:71–84.
37. Lange T, Gunther C, Kohler T, et al. High levels of BAX, low levels of MRP-1, and high platelets are independent predictors of response to imatinib in myeloid blast crisis of CML. Blood 2003; 101:2152–2155.
38. Thomas J, Wang L, Clark RE, and Pirmohamed M. Active transport of imatinib into and out of cells: implications for drug resistance. Blood 2004; 104:3739–3745.
39. Crossman LC, Druker BJ, Deininger MW, Pirmohamed M, Wang L, Clark RE. hOCT 1 and resistance to imatinib. Blood 2005; 106:1133–1134; author reply 1134.
40. Marktel S, Marin D, Foot N, et al. Chronic myeloid leukemia in chronic phase respond-ing to imatinib: the occurrence of additional cytogenetic abnormalities predicts disease progression. Haematologica 2003; 88:260–267.
41. Mitelman F. The cytogenetic scenario of chronic myeloid leukemia. Leuk Lymphoma 11 Suppl 1993; 1:11–15.
42. Cortes JE, Talpaz M, Giles F, et al. Prognostic significance of cytogenetic clonal evolution in patients with chronic myelogenous leukemia on imatinib mesylate therapy. Blood 2003; 101:3794–3800.
43. Fioretos T, Strombeck B, Sandberg T, et al. Isochromosome 17q in blast crisis of chronic myeloid leukemia and in other hematologic malignancies is the result of clustered breakpoints in 17p11 and is not associated with coding TP53 mutations. Blood 1999; 94:225–232.
44. Schutte J, Opalka B, Becher R, et al. Analysis of the p53 gene in patients with isochromo-some 17q and Ph1-positive or -negative myeloid leukemia. Leuk Res 1993; 17:533–539.
45. Jennings BA, Mills KI. c-myc locus amplification and the acquisition of trisomy 8 in the evolution of chronic myeloid leukaemia. Leuk Res 1998; 22:899–903.
46. Virtaneva K, Wright FA, Tanner SM, et al. Expression profiling reveals fundamental biological differences in acute myeloid leukemia with isolated trisomy 8 and normal cytogenetics. Proc Natl Acad Sci USA 2001; 98:1124–1129.
47. Wendel HG, de Stanchina E, Cepero E, et al. Loss of p53 impedes the antileukemic response to BCR-ABL inhibition. Proc Natl Acad Sci USA 2006; 103:7444–7449.
48. Yamamoto M, Kakihana K, Kurosu T, Murakami N, Miura O. Clonal evolution with inv(11)(p15q22) and NUP98/DDX10 fusion gene in imatinib-resistant chronic myelogen-ous leukemia. Cancer Genet Cytogenet 2005; 157:104–108.
49. Arai Y, Hosoda F, Kobayashi H, et al. The inv(11)(p15q22) chromosome translocation of de novo and therapy-related myeloid malignancies results in fusion of the nucleoporin gene, NUP98, with the putative RNA helicase gene, DDX10. Blood 1997; 89:3936–3944.
50. Donato NJ, Wu JY, Stapley J, et al. BCR-ABL independence and LYN kinase overexpres-sion in chronic myelogenous leukemia cells selected for resistance to STI571. Blood 2003; 101:690–698.
51. Hughes TP, Kaeda J, Branford S, et al. Frequency of major molecular responses to imatinib or interferon alfa plus cytarabine in newly diagnosed chronic myeloid leuke-mia. N Engl J Med 2003; 349:1423–1432.
52. Peng B, Hayes M, Resta D, et al. Pharmacokinetics and pharmacodynamics of imatinib in a phase I trial with chronic myeloid leukemia patients. J Clin Oncol 2004; 22:935–942.
53. Kantarjian HM, Talpaz M, O'Brien S, et al. Dose escalation of imatinib mesylate can overcome resistance to standard-dose therapy in patients with chronic myelogenous leukemia. Blood 2003; 101:473–475.
54. Zonder JA, Pemberton P, Brandt H, Mohamed AN, Schiffer CA. The effect of dose increase of imatinib mesylate in patients with chronic or accelerated phase chronic myelogenous leukemia with inadequate hematologic or cytogenetic response to initial treatment. Clin Cancer Res 2003; 9:2092–2097.
55. O'Brien S, Tefferi A, Valent P. Chronic myelogenous leukemia and myeloproliferative disease. Hematology (Am Soc Hematol Educ Program) 2004; 146–162.
56. Nicolini FE, Corm S, Le QH, et al. Mutation status and clinical outcome of 89 imatinib mesylate-resistant chronic myelogenous leukemia patients: a retrospective analysis from the French intergroup of CML (Fi(phi)-LMC GROUP). Leukemia 2006; 20:1061–1066.

57. Kantarjian H, Giles F, Wunderle L, et al. Nilotinib in imatinib-resistant CML and Philadelphia chromosome-positive ALL. N Engl J Med 2006; 354:2542–2551.
58. Mestan J, Weisberg E, Cowan-Jacob SW, et al. AMN107: In vitro profile of a new inhibitor of the tyrosine kinase activity of Bcr-Abl. Blood 2004; 104:546a.
59. Weisberg E, Manley PW, Breitenstein W, et al. Characterization of AMN107, a selective inhibitor of native and mutant Bcr-Abl. Cancer Cell 2005; 7:129–141.
60. Lombardo LJ, Lee FY, Chen P, et al. Discovery of N-(2-Chloro-6-methyl- phenyl)-2-(6-(4-(2-hydroxyethyl)-piperazin-1-yl)-2-methylpyrimidin-4-ylamino)thiazole-5-carboxamide (BMS-354825), a Dual Src/Abl Kinase Inhibitor with Potent Antitumor Activity in Preclinical Assays. J Med Chem 2004; 47:6658–6661.
61. Tokarski JS, Newitt JA, Chang CY, et al. The structure of Dasatinib (BMS-354825) bound to activated ABL kinase domain elucidates its inhibitory activity against imatinib-resistant ABL mutants. Cancer Res 2006; 66:5790–5797.
62. Shah NP, Tran C, Lee FY, Chen P, Norris D, Sawyers CL. Overriding imatinib resistance with a novel ABL kinase inhibitor. Science 2004; 305:399–401.
63. Talpaz M, Shah NP, Kantarjian H, et al. Dasatinib in imatinib-resistant Philadelphia chromosome-positive leukemias. N Engl J Med 2006; 354:2531–2541.
64. Huron DR, Gorre ME, Kraker AJ, Sawyers CL, Rosen N, Moasser MM. A novel pyrido-pyrimidine inhibitor of Abl kinase is a picomolar inhibitor of Bcr-abl-driven K562 cells and is effective against STI571-resistant Bcr-abl mutants. ClinCancer Res 2003; 9: 1267–1273.
65. La Rosee P, Corbin AS, Stoffregen EP, Deininger MW, Druker BJ. Activity of the Bcr-Abl kinase inhibitor PD180970 against clinically relevant Bcr-Abl isoforms that cause resistance to imatinib mesylate (Gleevec, STI571). Cancer Res 2002; 62:7149–7153.
66. Nagar B, Bornmann WG, Pellicena P, et al. Crystal structures of the kinase domain of c-Abl in complex with the small molecule inhibitors PD173955 and imatinib (STI-571). Cancer Res 2002; 62:4236–4243.
67. von Bubnoff N, Veach DR, Miller WT, et al. Inhibition of wild-type and mutant bcr-abl by pyrido-pyrimidine-type small molecule kinase inhibitors. Cancer Res 2003; 63: 6395–6404.
68. Wolff NC, Veach DR, Tong WP, Bornmann WG, Clarkson B, Ilaria RL. Jr. PD166326, a novel tyrosine kinase inhibitor, has greater antileukemic activity than imatinib mesylate in a murine model of chronic myeloid leukemia. Blood 2005; 105:3995–4003.
69. Golas JM, Arndt K, Etienne C, et al. SKI-606, a 4-anilino-3-quinolinecarbonitrile dual inhibitor of Src and Abl kinases, is a potent antiproliferative agent against chronic myelogenous leukemia cells in culture and causes regression of K562 xenografts in nude mice. Cancer Res 2003; 63:375–381.
70. Kimura S, Naito H, Segawa H, et al. NS-187, a potent and selective dual Bcr-Abl/Lyn tyrosine kinase inhibitor, is a novel agent for imatinib-resistant leukemia. Blood 2005; 106:3948–3954.
71. Gumireddy K, Baker SJ, Cosenza SC, et al. A non-ATP-competitive inhibitor of *BCR-ABL* overrides imatinib resistance. Proc Natl Acad Sci U S A 2005; 102:1992–1997.
72. Adrian FJ, Ding Q, Sim T, et al. Allosteric inhibitors of Bcr-abl-dependent cell proliferation. Nat Chem Biol 2006; 2:95–102.
73. Carter TA, Wodicka LM, Shah NP, et al. Inhibition of drug-resistant mutants of ABL, KIT, and EGF receptor kinases. Proc Natl Acad Sci USA 2005; 102:11011–11016.
74. Azam M, Latek RR, Daley GQ. Mechanisms of autoinhibition and STI-571/imatinib resistance revealed by mutagenesis of *BCR-ABL*. Cell 2003; 112:831–843.
75. O'Hare T, Pollock R, Stoffregen EP, et al. Inhibition of wild-type and mutant Bcr-Abl by AP23464, a potent ATP-based oncogenic protein kinase inhibitor: Implications for CML. Blood 2004; 104:2532–2539.
76. Azam M, Nardi V, Shakespeare WC, et al. Activity of dual SRC-ABL inhibitors highlights the role of *BCR/ABL* kinase dynamics in drug resistance. Proc Natl Acad Sci USA 2006; 103:9244–9249.
77. Bradeen HA, Eide CA, O'Hare T, et al. Comparison of imatinib, dasatinib (BMS-354825), and nilotinib (AMN107) in an n-ethyl-n-nitrosourea (ENU)-based mutagenesis screen: high efficacy of drug combinations. Blood 2006; 108:2332–2338.

78. Burgess MR, Skaggs BJ, Shah NP, Lee FY, Sawyers CL. Comparative analysis of two clinically active *BCR-ABL* kinase inhibitors reveals the role of conformation-specific binding in resistance. Proc Natl Acad Sci USA 2005; 102:3395–3400.

79. von Bubnoff N, Manley PW, Mestan J, Sanger J, Peschel C, Duyster J. Bcr-Abl resistance screening predicts a limited spectrum of point mutations to be associated with clinical resistance to the Abl kinase inhibitor nilotinib (AMN107). Blood 2006; 108:1328–1333.

80. Holyoake T, Jiang X, Eaves C, Eaves A. Isolation of a highly quiescent subpopulation of primitive leukemic cells in chronic myeloid leukemia. Blood 1999; 94:2056–2064.

81. Bhatia R, Holtz M, Niu N, et al. Persistence of malignant hematopoietic progenitors in chronic myelogenous leukemia patients in complete cytogenetic remission following imatinib mesylate treatment. Blood 2003; 101:4701–4707.

82. Graham SM, Jorgensen HG, Allan E, et al. Primitive, quiescent, Philadelphia-positive stem cells from patients with chronic myeloid leukemia are insensitive to STI571 in vitro. Blood 2002; 99:319–325.

83. Chu S, Xu H, Shah NP, et al. Detection of *BCR-ABL* kinase mutations in CD34+ cells from chronic myelogenous leukemia patients in complete cytogenetic remission on imatinib mesylate treatment. Blood 2005; 105:2093–2098.

84. Corbin AS, La Rosee P, Stoffregen EP, Druker BJ, Deininger MW. Several Bcr-Abl kinase domain mutants associated with imatinib mesylate resistance remain sensitive to imatinib. Blood 2003; 101:4611–4614.

8 Immunotherapy of Chronic Myeloid Leukemia

Monica Bocchia and Francesco Lauria

Department of Hematology, Siena University, Siena, Italy

INTRODUCTION

Imatinib has become standard therapy for all phases of chronic myeloid leukemia (CML). However, data generated by monitoring several thousands of patients worldwide suggest that although imatinib is highly active against the differentiated mass of CML cells, it probably fails to eradicate all residual leukemia cells, even in the best responders. This is supported by several lines of evidence: (*i*) despite the fact that more than 80% of previously untreated patients achieve a complete cytogenetic remission (CCgR), only a minority of patients remain durably negative when tested by real-time quantitative polymerase chain reaction (RT-PCR) for *BCR-ABL* transcripts (1); (*ii*) even patients treated with imatinib who achieve a complete molecular response (CMolR) usually return to Philadelphia (Ph)-positivity if the drug is stopped (2); and (*iii*) studies performed in vitro suggest that primitive Ph-positive progenitors or stem cells are relatively insensitive to imatinib (3) and the persistence of *BCR-ABL*-positive precursors in complete cytogenetic response (CCyR) patients, despite continued imatinib therapy, has been recently documented (4). At least theoretically, any amount of residual disease under imatinib treatment could provide the basis for the emergence of Ph-positive sub-clones bearing mutations in the *BCR-ABL* kinase domain, which are associated with various degrees of resistance to this agent (5). For all these reasons recent CML guidelines recommend that alternative strategies should be considered in early chronic phase (CP) patients with suboptimal response or failure to adequate imatinib (6). Less straightforward is the management of residual "molecular" disease found in a great majority of patients. At present, these patients usually continue to receive standard doses of imatinib, and their response is monitored by RT-PCR and cytogenetics. Although we do not yet know the impact on survival of such minimal residual disease (MRD) (7), it appears prudent to develop specific additional therapies that could complete the excellent work of imatinib. The ultimate and ambitious aim of a supplementary treatment would be the attainment of a "true cure" of CML (eradication of all leukemia cells) instead of an "operational cure" (persistence of minimal amount of leukemia cells), which may be achieved with imatinib alone. One such strategy is to exploit the fact that CML is a disease known to be susceptible to immune attack. The most striking proof of this is the fact that until now, a "cure" (defined as continuous negativity for *BCR-ABL* by PCR) for CML patients is probably achieved only by the graft-versus-leukemia (GvL) effect following allogeneic stem cell transplantation or donor lymphocytes infusion (8), although it remains formally unproven that undetectability of *BCR-ABL* is equivalent to eradication of the malignant clone. Although the GvL effect is to a great extent due to major and minor HLA mismatches between donors and recipients, some experimental data suggest that CML-specific donor T lymphocytes could be the key to long-term control or even eradication of residual leukemia cells (9). Additionally, the activity of interferon-α (IFN-α), a biological modifier widely used for CML in the pre-imatinib era, could be partly due to an immune-mediated effect, and a possible role of this agent in the context of MRD surviving imatinib will be discussed. CML offers a unique opportunity to test the efficacy and feasibility of immunotherapeutic strategies, as currently most patients achieve very pronounced responses furnishing an ideal situation for immunotherapy in a disease known to be responsive in principle to immune attack. Immunotherapy approaches currently under evaluation include active specific immunotherapies (vaccines) and nonspecific immunotherapies [IFN-α, interleukin-2 (IL-2), granulocyte-macrophage colony stimulating factor (GM-CSF), and other immunostimulators].

ACTIVE SPECIFIC IMMUNOTHERAPY: VACCINES

As a general concept a "therapeutic antitumor vaccine" refers to the subcutaneous administration of a tumor-specific antigen with the intent to induce an active and possibly long-lasting humoral and/or cellular immune response able to eliminate tumor cells harboring the putative antigen. Many years of disappointing clinical results with antitumor vaccines against different types of advanced solid tumors has taught tumor immunologists that the best setting for effective immunotherapy is the situation of MRD (10). In CML, like in other tumors, the ideal vaccine candidate would be an antigen expressed only in tumor cells, but common to all patients. It should be highly immunogenic and should be essential for tumor cell survival, and thus not susceptible to mutation or deletion. Several CML antigens have been identified as potential targets for an anti-CML vaccine strategy (Fig. 1), and different approaches at different stages of development are now under evaluation for CML patients (Table 1).

True "Chronic Myeloid Leukemia-Specific" Antigen Vaccines

The *BCR-ABL*—derived p210 protein and particularly the alternative b3a2 or b2a2 peptide epitope at its fusion point is the most obvious CML-specific target, and thus was first explored for a vaccine strategy. p210 is exclusive to the CML clone, and the sequences of amino acids contained in the b3a2 and b2a2 junctional regions represent unique tumor-specific determinants, which can be exploited for an immunological attack against the tumor cell (11). Recent data support the hypothesis that peptides binding HLA with moderate-to-high affinity are capable of stimulating T-cells after natural processing and cell surface presentation within the cleft of the appropriate HLA molecule. Within the p210 b3a2 breakpoint sequence, five junctional peptides were found to be capable of binding to certain HLA class I and class II molecules and were shown to elicit in vitro a specific T-cell response both in normal donors (12) and in CML patients (13). After these initial observations, p210 b3a2 breakpoint peptides have also been shown to induce cytotoxic T cells (CTLs) and CD4+ cells able to induce cell death and to inhibit proliferation of leukemia cells, respectively (14). Finally, the relevance of these peptides as truly immunogenic tumor antigens has been confirmed by their capability to be "endogenously" presented within class I and class II molecules

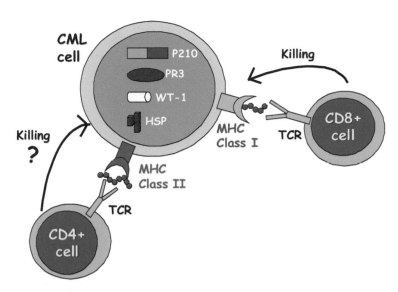

FIGURE 1 Tumor-associated antigens that are now under evaluation for vaccine therapy in chronic myeloid leukemia (CML) (bcr–abl-derived P210; myeloblastin (PR-3), Wilm's Tumor protein (WT-1); Heat shock proteins. In CML cells, peptides derived by these antigens may be presented on the cell surface both through the MHC class I and class II pathway, thus inducing both CD8+ and CD4+ T cell antitumor response. *Abbreviations*: CML, chronic myeloid leukemia; MHC, major histocompatibility complex; TCR, T cell receptor; HSP, heat shock protein.

of CML blasts and CML dendritic cells (DCs) (15,16). All these findings provided powerful scientific support for a b3a2-breakpoint peptides vaccine approach.

"Native" BCR-ABL *Breakpoint-Derived Vaccines*
The first phase I/II vaccine trials employing a mixture of five or more b3a2-derived peptides plus the immunological adjuvant QS-21 included CML patients in CP during conventional treatment (17,18). These trials have documented for the first time the capability of CML breakpoint peptides to elicit peptide-specific CD8+ and CD4+ T cell responses in CML patients with a relatively large tumor burden. However, despite some decrease in the proportion of Ph-positive metaphases observed in some patients, a clear relationship between clinical responses and vaccination could not be established in these studies.

As it is more likely that effective vaccination strategies will target patients with MRD, a similar phase II b3a2-derived peptide vaccine multicenter trial was conducted at the Department of Hematology in Siena, Italy, and included patients with b3a2-positive CML, proper HLA restriction, and a major or complete cytogenetic response to imatinib or IFN-α (19). The vaccine (CMLVAX100) consisted of five b3a2 breakpoint-derived peptides plus QS-21. To increase peptide immunogenicity and possibly antitumor effect, low doses of GM-CSF as co-immunoadjuvant were also included. Sixteen CML patients with stable cytogenetic or molecular residual disease for at least six months on treatment with imatinib or IFN-α were vaccinated. After six planned vaccinations of 10 patients on imatinib, all 10 patients improved their responses. In particular, five of nine patients with cytogenetic disease before the vaccination reached CCyR and 4/9 reduced the

TABLE 1 Current Approaches for Immunotherapy of Chronic Myeloid Leukemia

Antigen	Method of delivery	Advantages	Disadvantages	Stage of development
Peptides				
CML-specific b3a2 and b2a2 bcr–abl fusion "native" peptides b3a2 and b2a2 fusion "heteroclitic" peptides	Subcutaneous vaccine with adjuvants	Specific targeting Simple, rapid, and inexpensive production Unlimited availability Best GMP compliance Easy to monitor response	Certain HLA type may have better response than others Single Ag targeting may lead to tumor escape mechanism	Phase II
Tumor associated PR3-derived peptides WT-1-derived peptides	Subcutaneous vaccine with adjuvants	Specific targeting[a] Simple, rapid, and inexpensive production[a] Unlimited availability[a] Best GMP compliance[a] Easy to monitor response[a]	Ags also expressed on other tissues	Preclinical and phase I and II studies
CML-derived material HSP complexes	Subcutaneous vaccine	All CML Ags available Specific mechanism for uptake	Complex preparation for individual patient	Phase II

				Limited vaccinations depending on initial yield of HSP; Difficult to monitor specific response	Pilot and pre-clinical studies
Cell-based	Ph-positive DC loaded with CML-derived peptides or genetically modified CML cell lines	Subcutaneous vaccine	All tumor Ags available; Powerful inducers of immune response (DCs)	Complex preparation for individual patients (DCs); Limited availability of vaccine; Ph-positive DCs are less efficient APCs; Difficult to monitor specific responses	Pilot and pre-clinical studies
Non specific immuno-stimulators	IFN-α; IL-2; GM-CSF	Subcutaneous	Induce a variety of immune responses against CML cells	Require low tumor burden; Can be associated with toxicity	In addition to imatinib in some phase II studies

[a] All these advantages are for tumor specificity.

Abbreviations: Ags, antigens; APC, antigen presenting cell; DC, dendritic cell; CML, chronic myeloid leukemia; GMP, good manufacturing practise; HLA, human leukocyte antigen; HSP, heat shock protein; IFN-α, interferon-α; IL-2, interleukin-2; GM-CSF, granulocyte-macrophage colony stimulating factor.

TABLE 2 Disease Response after Vaccinations with CMLVAX100 plus QS-21 and Granulocyte-Macrophage Colony Stimulating Factor: Updated Results of the Phase II Clinical Trial

Disease status at enrollment (time 0)		Response after six CMLVAX100 (3 mo)		Response after three additional boosts (18 mo)		Response after six additional boosts (32 mo)
		23 patients		11 patients		6 patients
Major/minor cytogenetic response	10	6 CCyR[a] (4 CMR[b]) 2 improved 2 stable disease	8	5 CCyR 2 maintaining CMolR 1 improved	6	1 CCyR 1 >1 log improved 3 CMolR 1 relapse (never CMolR)
Complete cytogenetic response	10	7>1 log improved (2 CMolR) 3 stable disease	3	1 improved (CMolR) 1 maintaining CMolR 1 CCyR	—	—
Hematologic response	3	3 no response	—	—	—	—

Note: At enrollment, the median time of imatinib treatment and the median time of established residual disease were 24 months (range, 12–50) and 12 months (range, 6–33), respectively.
[a]Complete cytogenetic response defined as absence of t(9;22)(q34;q21) in at least 30 metaphases.
[b]Complete molecular response defined as: BCR-ABL transcript undetectable by nested RT-PCR or BCR-ABL/Abl ratio <0.001 or BCR-ABL/β_2 microglobulin ratio <0.00001).
Abbreviations: CCyR, complete cytogenetic response; CMolR, complete molecular response.

percentage of residual Ph-positive cells. Furthermore, 3/5 patients that reached CCyR achieved molecular negativity. One imatinib patient vaccinated while in CCyR experienced a half-log reduction of his residual disease. Of six patients on IFN-alpha, all but one had a further reduction of residual disease, with two reaching CCyR. The clinical responses were associated with a peptide-specific immune response. After six vaccinations, peptide-specific delayed type hypersensitivity (DTH) skin reactions were seen in 10/16 patients, and a peptide-specific CD4+ T cell proliferation in vitro was measured in 13/14 patients studied. The predominant immunological effect produced by the vaccine appeared to be mediated by a 25 amino acid peptide, which contains several epitopes for different HLA class II molecules, some of which were newly identified along the study. Much less evident was the immunological effect of the short peptides included in the vaccine, as only few peptide-specific CTLs were documented. The lack of a CTL response may be a consequence of the low affinity of binding of the short CML peptides to proper HLA molecules, or simply due to the use of in vitro assays not sensitive enough to detect a weak but relevant cytotoxic response. The great majority of the patients experienced no toxicity to this vaccine other than mild local pain and redness and itching at the site of vaccination. No systemic adverse events and no severe adverse events have been recorded (19). At present, a total of 25 b3a2-CML patients with various degrees of cytogenetically and/or molecularly defined MRD persisting after a median time of two years of imatinib treatment have entered this trial. A further reduction of MRD (including some CMR) after vaccinations has been observed in about 65% of this extended series of patients. The updated results of 23/25 evaluable patients are summarized in Table 2. However, the overall clinical benefit of inducing a long lasting peptide-specific immune response in imatinib treated patients has yet to be demonstrated. Only a randomized phase III trial, planned in the near future, will define the role of this vaccine approach in preventing disease recurrence.

In the initial studies no peptide sequence suitable for a similar vaccine strategy was found across the b2a2 fusion point, the alternative p210 breakpoint that is found in about 40% of CML patients. Only recently, some peptide sequences encompassing the b2a2 breakpoint were found capable of binding to certain HLA class II molecules and to elicit an immune response in vitro (20). Hence, a similar immunotherapeutic approach employing a 25-mer b2a2-derived peptide and GM-CSF as adjuvant for b2a2 CML patients with persisting MRD on imatinib treatment is now under investigation.

Synthetic (Heteroclitic) bcr-abl–Derived Peptide Vaccines

As previously discussed, "native" amino acid sequences reliably elicit bcr-abl peptide-specific CD4+ immune responses while cytotoxic CD8+ responses are weak and rarely observed, probably due to low binding affinity of the natural CML peptides to HLA class I molecules. Although a role of CD4+ cells as direct mediators of an antitumor effect has recently been suggested (21), it is a generally held belief that cytotoxic T-cell responses are required to induce reproducible antileukemic activity. One strategy to overcome the poor immunogenicity of BCR-ABL peptides to cytotoxic CD8 cells is to design synthetic analogous peptides that may be more immunogenic (22). Such peptide analogues could generate an immune response that not only recognizes the immunizing epitopes, but also cross-reacts with the original native peptides; this is known as a heteroclitic response. In this context, a pilot study was initiated at Memorial Sloan Kettering Cancer Center to determine whether heteroclitic peptides analogous to HLA A0201 binding bcr-abl sequences could stimulate an immune response to the native HLA A0201 bcr-abl sequence in CML patients with a response to imatinib therapy. Peptides were mixed with Montanide adjuvant, and GM-CSF was used as additional stimulant. Immune responses were measured after five biweekly vaccinations. So far this study included 11 CML patients with MRD on imatinib. Preliminary data show that in 8/8 patients tested vaccination induced an immunologic response to the analogous peptides as well as to the native peptides, and in 5/11 patients a reduction of MRD levels was also observed (23).

Shared Tumor Antigen Peptide Vaccines

Another active-specific immunotherapy with potential antitumor effect in CML relies on the use of intracellular proteins other than p210. In fact a number of self proteins are aberrantly overexpressed in CML and other tumor cells while being expressed at low levels in normal lineages and thus may function as targets for directed immunotherapy of residual disease. As in the case of p210, despite the intracellular location of these proteins, short peptides produced by their cellular processing can be presented on the cell surface within the cleft of HLA molecules and in this form they can be recognized by T cells. Several peptide vaccines derived from such proteins have reached the stage of clinical development in CML patients.

Proteinase-3-Derived Peptide Vaccines

Proteinase-3 (PR3) or myeloblastin is a 26-kd neutral serine protease normally expressed in hematopoietic tissues and highly expressed in myeloid haematological malignancies. PR1, an HLA-A2.1-restricted nonamer peptide derived from PR3, has been identified as a tumor-specific antigen in myeloid leukemia. Cytotoxic T lymphocytes recognizing PR1 that are capable of lysing fresh leukemia cells have been detected in CML patients and have been implicated in the clearance of malignant cells in patients treated with IFN-α or stem cell transplantation (SCT) (24). Vaccinations of PR1 peptide in Montanide were administered subcutaneously every three weeks for a total of three doses to 10 CML patients not responding to treatment or with relapsed disease (25). Preliminary reports indicate that a significant increase in PR1 CTLs was evident in about 60% of vaccinated patients. Clinical responses included one CCyR and stable disease with some hematologic improvement in three cases. Responses were correlated with the induction of PR1-specific CTLs with a central memory (CCR7+) phenotype, indicative of a self-renewing population (26). However, there is good evidence that imatinib therapy down-regulates PR3 expression in CML cells and this could potentially reduce the antitumor activity of this approach (27). In fact, especially in the context of MRD persisting on prolonged treatment with imatinib, leukemic cells may harbor only minimal amounts of PR3 that are insufficient for proper PR1 peptide HLA presentation. Consequently, PR1-specific CTLs induced with the vaccinations may be unable to recognize and clear residual cells due to an inadequate number of PR-1–HLA complexes on the cell surface. One way to circumvent this problem could be to stop imatinib treatment temporarily after immunization with PR-1 vaccine in order to "restore" the PR3 content of the residual CML cells and allow their recognition and elimination by PR-1 specific CTLs.

Wilm's Tumor Protein-Derived Peptide Vaccines

Another candidate for a peptide vaccine approach in CML is the Wilm's tumor protein (WT-1)—a self protein overexpressed in most human leukemias, including CML and some solid tumors, but rarely present in normal cells (28). Recent studies have identified WT-1-specific CTLs in CML patients (29). Importantly, in vitro models have demonstrated that WT-1-specific CTLs deplete leukemic but not normal CD34+ stem cells (30) suggesting that they may be effective in eradicating the quiescent stem cells present in MRD. Additionally, intravenous injection of human T cells transduced with a WT-1 T-cell receptor into NOD/SCID mice harbouring human leukemia cells resulted in leukemia elimination (31).

Promising clinical results were observed in patients with acute myeloid leukemias and myelodysplastic syndromes after vaccinations with WT-1-derived peptides and Montanide ISA51 or GM-CSF as adjuvants (32). A significant correlation was observed between an increase in the frequencies of WT1-specific CTLs after WT1 vaccination and clinical responses (32). However, similar peptide vaccination studies have not yet been published in CML patients with MRD.

Chronic Myeloid Leukemia Cell-Derived Multi-Antigen Vaccines

Heat Shock Protein Vaccines

Heat shock proteins (HSPs) are ubiquitous protective intracellular molecules induced by cellular stress, which act as chaperones for peptides. HSPs isolated from tumor cells carry an array of tumor-specific peptides capable of inducing immune responses. In fact, purified HSP–peptide complexes have been demonstrated to activate CD8+ and CD4+ lymphocytes to induce innate immune responses, including natural killer (NK) cell activation, cytokine secretion, and induce maturation of DCs (33). In a phase I trial, vaccinations with patient-specific autologous leukocyte-derived HSP70 peptide complexes were given to 20 CML patients who had cytogenetic or molecular evidence of disease despite ongoing treatment with imatinib (34). In each patient entering this study, HSP70 was purified from the leukapheresed peripheral blood mononuclear cells and administered in eight-week intervals as intradermal injections without immunological adjuvant. The vaccine produced no adverse effects and was associated with a reduction in Ph-positive cells and/or *BCR-ABL* expression in 13/20 patients. Immunologic responses, measured as increased IFN-γ expression in T cells against pre-vaccination leukocyte targets, were observed in 9/16 patients analyzed (34). A significant correlation between clinical responses and immunologic responses was observed. Phase II clinical trials are currently underway.

Other Vaccine Candidates

Although not yet tested in clinical trials, several other molecules that are either CML-specific or preferentially expressed by CML cells are under evaluation as potential targets for immunotherapy. These include CML66 and CML28 tumor-associated antigens found both in leukemias and in a variety of solid tumor cell lines, but not in normal hematopoietic tissue (35). Other potential immunotherapeutic targets in CML are survivin, an antiapoptotic molecule up-regulated in CML cells (36), telomerase, thought to be involved in disease progression and potentially linked to imatinib resistance (37), and RHAMM/CD168 expressed in about 83% of CML cells and able to mediate a specific T cell response in CML patients (38).

Cell-Based Vaccines

An additional approach of inducing a CML-specific immune attack against MRD exploits the capacity of DCs to efficiently process and present antigens, which leads to effective sensitization of naïve T lymphocytes (39). Human DCs can be obtained from CD34+ bone marrow cells and from human peripheral monocytes in the presence of cytokine combinations. As the majority of CML DCs carry t(9;22), the immune response induced by an "unprimed DCs"-based vaccine approach relies on presentation of leukemic antigens inherently expressed by the leukemic DC. Autologous *BCR-ABL*-positive DCs have been safely used for vaccinations in CP patients with an insufficient response to imatinib and have been shown to induce CML-specific T-cell responses in association with a decrease in tumor cell burden/circulating *BCR-ABL*-positive cells (40). The feasibility of this patient-specific vaccine approach in the setting of MRD after imatinib needs further evaluation, as imatinib treatment dramatically reduces Ph-positive DCs and it could be difficult to generate an adequate amount for vaccination. Additionally, the immunologic efficiency may be reduced if imatinib adversely affected DC function (41,42). An alternative approach is to generate more efficient targeted immune responses by loading (or "priming") Ph-positive or Ph-negative DCs with tumor-specific antigens (i.e., *BCR-ABL*, PR3 or WT-1 derived peptides, and HSPs or autologous tumor lysates). In this setting, peptide-specific immune responses, but no clinical improvement, were observed in three patients vaccinated with b3a2 fusion peptide-primed DCs (43). A different cell-based vaccine approach is underway in a pilot clinical trial in which irradiated K562 cells genetically modified to secrete GM-CSF (K562/GM-CSF) are administered subcutaneously to CML patients undergoing therapy with imatinib (44).

NONSPECIFIC IMMUNOTHERAPY

Interferon-α

IFN-α has been a standard therapy for CP CML for nearly two decades. The introduction of imatinib has replaced its role as first line agent, but IFN-α could play a key role in modulating a nonspecific immune-mediated effect toward MRD persisting during imatinib therapy. Several immunologic effects of IFN-α have been documented, including increased expression of adhesion molecules, and enhanced antigen presentation and generation of highly active monocyte-derived DCs (45). Nevertheless, it is still unclear as to which effect is precisely responsible for its antileukemic activity. Recently, the presence of PR3-specific CTLs has been documented in IFN-α-treated patients, but not in imatinib-treated patients. This suggests that IFN-α may enhance the induction of "natural" anti-PR3 CTLs, thus modulating a direct immune-mediated antitumor effect against CML cells (27). Indirect evidence of an underlying immune control of leukemic cells mediated by IFN-α is the fact that some patients maintain CCyR without recurrence of disease for many years after discontinuation of the drug despite persistence of molecular MRD (46). Furthermore, it has recently been observed that 4/7 patients previously exposed to IFN-α maintained CMR for 8 to 13 months after discontinuation of imatinib (47). All these premises provide a novel rationale for employing low doses of IFN-α as promoter of an innate antileukemic immune response both in patients with MRD persisting during imatinib treatment as well as in those patients who have to or wish to stop imatinib after achieving low levels of residual disease.

Interleukin-2

The T-cell growth factor IL-2 can induce both tumor-specific CTLs and memory T cell proliferation that may help in maintaining CTLs mediated antitumor activity over time. Before the advent of imatinib, low dose IL-2 had been used as a therapy for advanced CML with little clinical benefit (48). Today, IL-2 could play a renovated role in boosting and maintaining immune responses induced by CML-specific immunotherapies, once imatinib has established a state of MRD.

Granulocyte-Macrophage Colony Stimulating Factor

Subcutaneous low dose GM-CSF is capable of recruiting and enhancing the activity of local antigen presenting cells, and this myeloid growth factor has been employed as an immunological adjuvant for antitumor vaccination in CML (19). GM-CSF may also improve the activity of IFN-α as primary therapy for CML (49), and a recent randomized study has explored the combination of GM-CSF and IFN-α in addition to high doses of imatinib as front line treatment for CML patients (50). The GM-CSF plus IFN-α arm of this study appeared to have a trend for improved CCyR and MMR rates at 12 months over the IFN-α only arm, although longer follow-up is required. Overall these data suggest that GM-CSF may enhance the activity of IFN-α against CML cells by boosting nonspecific antitumor immune effects. GM-CSF should also be evaluated in the context of MRD persisting on imatinib treatment.

PERSPECTIVES

As of now there are several immunotherapeutic strategies that could be proposed to a CML patient with MRD during standard imatinib treatment. From a practical point of view, the ideal candidate for an immune approach should meet several requirements: first, it should be an agent that specifically and effectively targets only residual leukemia cells; secondly, it should be well tolerated; and thirdly, it should be one single agent for all patients, preferably not too expensive and too laborious to produce and with an immune activity easy to monitor. On the basis of these considerations, *BCR-ABL*-based peptide vaccination appears to be a widely feasible strategy, with convincing immunologic data and with promising clinical effects. Similarly, PR3- and WT-1-based peptide vaccines appear to be practicable approaches, but clinical data especially in the context of MRD are still very limited. In contrast, strategies based on the preparation of a specific vaccine for each single patient (i.e., HSP vaccine and DC-based vaccines) while promising in terms of potential immunologic and clinical benefit may be less feasible due to the more difficult logistics of vaccine production. For example, in cases of HSPs-based vaccines, there may be a limited availability of vaccine due to a suboptimal HSPs yield from the leukapheresis performed at diagnosis. Likewise, the preparation of a vaccine with Ph-positive DCs may be difficult when the CML burden is low due to imatinib treatment, whereas on the other hand the isolation of Ph-positive DCs at diagnosis could result in cells with less immunogenic activity (42). Of the nonspecific immunotherapeutic approaches, low doses of IFN-α may be most effective for residual disease and should be considered for MRD-positive CML patients.

CONCLUSION

The outcome of patients with CML has improved enormously since the introduction of imatinib. Despite this it appears that in most of even the best responders imatinib fails to eradicate all leukemia cells, a situation sometimes referred to as "functional cure." It is conceivable that more potent tyrosine kinase inhibitors, such as nilotinib and dasatinib, may have a more profound effect on leukemic stem cells. However, in vitro data show that dasatinib at least is not capable of killing quiescent cells, suggesting that the situation may not fundamentally differ from imatinib, with the majority of patients remaining MRD-positive. Although the impact on survival from such residual disease remains to be determined with longer follow-up, a continued search is warranted for alternative approaches aimed at eradicating the disease. Preliminary clinical data as well as pre-clinical studies suggest that CML-specific immunotherapy and particularly CML-specific vaccines may represent an attractive tool to achieve this ambitious goal.

REFERENCES

1. Cortes J, Talpaz M, O'Brien S, et al. Molecular responses in patients with chronic myelogenous leukemia in chronic phase treated with imatinib mesylate. Clin Cancer Res 2005; 11(9):3425–3432.
2. Cortes J, O'Brien S, Kantarjian H. Discontinuation of imatinib therapy after achieving a molecular response. Blood 2004; 104(7):2204–2205.
3. Graham SM, Jorgensen HG, Allan E, et al. Primitive, quiescent, Philadelphia-positive stem cells from patients with chronic myeloid leukemia are insensitive to STI571 in vitro. Blood 2002; 99(1):319–325.
4. Bhatia R, Holtz M, Niu N, et al. Persistence of malignant hematopoietic progenitors in chronic myelogenous leukemia patients in complete cytogenetic remission following imatinib mesylate treatment. Blood 2003; 101(12):4701–4707.

5. Hochhaus A, Kreil S, Corbin AS, et al. Molecular and chromosomal mechanisms of resistance to imatinib (STI571) therapy. Leukemia 2002; 16(11):2190–2196.
6. Baccarani M, Saglio G, Goldman J, et al. Evolving concepts in the management of chronic myeloid leukemia. Recommendations from an expert panel on behalf of the European Leukemianet. Blood Epub May 2006.
7. Goldman J, Gordon M. Why do chronic myelogenous leukemia stem cells survive allogeneic stem cell transplantation or imatinib: does it really matter? Leukemia and Lymphoma 2006; 47(1):1–7.
8. Kolb HJ, Mittermuller J, Clemm C, et al. Donor leukocytes transfusions for treatment of recurrent chronic myelogenous leukemia in marrow transplant patients. Blood 1990; 76 (12):2462–2465.
9. Bleakley M, Riddel SR. Molecules and mechanism of the graft-versus-leukemia effect. Nat Rev Cancer 2004; 4(5):371–380.
10. Bocchia M, Bronte V, Colombo MP, et al. Antitumor vaccination: where we stand. Haematologica 2000; 85(11):1172–1206.
11. Bocchia M, Wentworth PA, Southwood S, et al. Specific binding of leukemia oncogene fusion protein peptides to HLA class I molecules. Blood 1995; 85(10):2680–2684.
12. Bocchia M, Korontsvit T, Xu Q, et al. Specific human cellular immunity to bcr-abl oncogene derived peptides. Blood 1996; 87(9):3587–3592.
13. Bosh GJ, Joosten AM, Kessler JH, et al. Recognition of *BCR-ABL* positive leukemia blast by human DC4+ T cells elicited by primary in vitro immunization with a *BCR-ABL* breakpoint peptide. Blood 1996; 88(9):3522–3527.
14. Mannering SI, McKenzie JL, Fearnley DB, et al. HLA-DR1-restricted bcr-abl (b3a2-specific CD4+ T lymphocytes respond to dendritic cells pulsed with b3a2 peptide and antigen-presenting cells exposed to b3a2 containing cell lysates. Blood 1997; 90(1):290–297.
15. Clark RE, Dodi AI, Hill SC, et al. Direct evidence that leukemic cells present HLA-associated immunogenic peptides derived from the *BCR-ABL* b3a2 fusion protein. Blood 2001; 98(10):2887–2893.
16. Yasukama M, Ohminami H, Kojima K, et al. HLA class II-restricted antigen presentation of endogenous bcr-abl fusion protein by chronic myelogenous leukemia-derived dendritic cells to CD4 (+) T lymphocytes. Blood 2001; 98(10):1498–1505.
17. Pinilla-Ibarz J, Cathcart K, Korontsvit T, et al. Vaccination of patients with chronic myelogenous leukemia with bcr-abl oncogene breakpoint fusion peptides generates specific immune response. Blood 2000; 95(5):1781–1787.
18. Cathcart K, Pinilla-Ibarz J, Korontsvit T, et al. A multivalent bcr-abl fusion peptide vaccination trial in patients with chronic myeloid leukemia. Blood 2003; 103(3):1037–1042.
19. Bocchia M, Gentili S, Abruzzese E, et al. Effect of a p210 multipeptide vaccine associated with imatinib or interferon in patients with chronic myeloid leukemia and persistent residual disease: a multicentre observational trial. Lancet 2005; 365: 657–662.
20. ten Bosch GJA, Kessler JH, Joosten AM, et al. A bcr-abl oncoprotein p210b2a2 fusion region sequence is recognized by HLA-DR2a restricted cytotoxic T lymphocytes and presented by HLA-DR matched cells transfected with an lib^{2a2} construct. Blood 1999; 94(3):1038–1045.
21. Lundin KU, Hofgaard PO, Omholt H, et al. Therapeutic effect of idiotype-specific CD4+ cells against B-cell lymphoma in the absence of anti-idiotypic antibodies. Blood 2003; 102(2):605–612.
22. Pinilla-Ibarz J, Korontsvit T, Zackhaleva V, et al. Synthetic peptide analogs derived from bcr/abl fusion proteins and the induction of heteroclitic human T cell responses. Hematologica 2005; 90(10):1324–1332.
23. Maslak PG, Dao T, Gupta S, et al. Pilot trial of a synthetic breakpoint peptide vaccine in patients with chronic myeloid leukemia (CML) and minimal disease. J Clin Oncol 2006; 24(18S):6514a.
24. Molldrem JJ, Lee PP, Wang C, et al. Evidence that specific T lymphocytes may participate in the elimination of chronic myelogenous leukemia. Nat Med 2000; 6(9):1018–1023.

25. Qazilbash MH, Wieder E, Rios R, et al. Vaccination with the PR-1 leukemia associated antigen can induce complete remission in patients with myeloid leukemia, Blood (ASH annual meeting abstracts) 2004; 104:259a.
26. Wieder Ed, Kant S, Lu S, et al. PR-1 peptide vaccination of myeloid leukemia patients induces PR-1 specific CTL with high CCR7 expression. Blood (ASH annual meeting abstracts) 2003; 102:611a.
27. Burchert A, Wolf S, Schmidt M, et al. Interferon-alpha but not the ABL-kinase inhibitor imatinib (STI571), induces expression of myeloblastin and a specific T-cell response in chronic myeloid leukemia. Blood 2003; 101(1):259–264.
28. Menssen HD, Renkl HJ, Rodeck U, et al. Presence of Wilms' tumor gene (WT-1) transcript and the WT-1 nuclear protein in the majority of human acute leukemia. Leukemia 1997; 9(6): 1060–1067.
29. Bellantuono I, Gao L, Parry S, et al. Two distinct HLA-A0201-presented epitopes of the Wilms tumor antigen 1 can function as targets for leukemia-reactive CTL. Blood 2002; 100(10): 3835–3837.
30. Gao L, Bellantuono I, Elsasser A, et al. Selective elimination of leukemic CD34+ progenitor cells by cytotoxic T lymphocytes specific for WT1. Blood 2000; 95(7):2198–2203.
31. Xue SA, Gao L, Hart D, et al. Elimination of leukemia cells in NOD/SCID mice by WT1-TCR gene-transduced human T cells. Blood 2005; 106(9):3062–3067.
32. Oka Y, Tsuboi A, Taguchi T, et al. Induction of WT1 (Wilms' tumor gene)-specific cytotoxic T lymphocytes by WT1 peptide vaccine and the resultant cancer regression. Proc Nat Acad Sci USA 2004; 101(38):13885–13890.
33. Hoos A, Levey DL. Vaccination with heat shock protein–peptide complexes: from basic science to clinical applications. Expert Rev Vaccines 2003; 2(3):369–379.
34. Li Z, Qiao Y, Liu B, et al. Combination of imatinib mesylate with autologous leukocyte-derived heat shock protein and chronic myelogenous leukemia. Clin Cancer Res 2005; 11(12):4460–4468.
35. Greiner J, Ringhoffer M, Taniguchi M. Characterization of several leukemia-associated antigens inducing humoral immune responses in acute and chronic myeloid leukemia. Int J Cancer 2003; 106(2):224–231.
36. Carter BZ, Schober WD, McQueen T, et al. Regulation of surviving expression through bcr-abl/MAPK cascade: surviving as a therapeutic target in STI571 resistant CML cells. Blood (ASH annual meeting abstract) 2003; 102:651a.
37. Bakalova R, Ohba H, Zhelev Z, et al. Cross-talk between bcr-abl tyrosine kinase, protein kinase C and telomerase a potential reason for resistance to Glivec in chronic myelogenous leukemia. Biochem Pharmacol 2003; 66(10):1879–1884.
38. Greiner J, Li L, Giannopoulos K et al. Identification and characterization of epitopes of the receptor for hyaluronic acid-mediated motlity (RHAMM/CD168) recognized by CD8+ T cells of HLA-A2 positive patients with acute myelid leukemia. Blood (ASH annual meeting abstract) 2005, 106(3):2886a
39. Banchereau J, Steinman R. Dendritic cells and the control of immunity. Nature 1998; 392(6673):245–252.
40. Westermann J, Kopp J, van Lessen A, et al. Dendritic cells vaccination in BCR/ABL-positive chronic myeloid leukemia. Final results of a phase I/II study. Blood (ASH annual meeting abstracts) 2004; 104:2943a.
41. Wang H, Cheng F, Cuenca A, et al. Imatinib mesylate (STI-571) enhances antigen-presenting cell function and overcomes tumor-induced CD4+ T-cell tolerance. Blood 2005; 105(3):1135–1143.
42. Boissel N, Rousselot P, Raffoux F, et al. Imatinib mesylate minimally affects bcr-abl+ and normal monocyte-derived dendritic cells but strongly inhibits T cell expansion despite reciprocal dendritic cell-activation. J Leuk Biol 2006; 79(4):747–756.
43. Takahashi T, Tanaka Y, Nieda M, et al. Dendritic cell vaccination for patients with chronic myelogenous leukemia. Leuk Res 2003; 27(9):795–802.
44. Smith BD, Kasamon IL, Miller CB, et al. K562/GM-CSF vaccinations reduces tumor burden, including achieving molecular remissions, in chronic myeloid leukemia patients with residual disease on imatinib mesylate. J Clin Onc 2006; 24(18S):6509a.

45. Gabriele L, Borghi P, Rozera C, et al. IFN-α promotes the rapid differentiation of monocytes from patients with chronic myeloid leukemia into activated dendritic cells tuned to undergo full maturation after LPS treatment. Blood 2004; 103(3):980–987.
46. Mahon FX, Delbrel X, Cony-Makhoul P, et al. Follow-up of complete cytogenetic remission in patients with chronic myeloid leukemia after cessation of interferon alfa. J Clin Oncol 2002; 20(1):214–220.
47. Rosselot P, Huguet F, Cayuela JM, et al. Imatinib mesylate discontinuation in patients with chronic myelogenous leukemia in complete molecular remission for more than two years. Blood 2005 (ASH annual meeting abstract); 106:1001a.
48. Vey N, Blaise D, Lafage M, et al. Treatment of chronic myelogenous leukemia with interleukin-2 (IL-2): a phase II study in 21 patients. J Immunother 1999; 22(2):175–181.
49. Smith BD, Matsui WH, Murphy K, et al. GM-CSF improves activity of interferon as primary therapy for CML. Blood 2004 (ASH annual meeting abstract); 104:4678a.
50. Cortes J, Talpaz M, O'Brien S, et al. A randomized trial of high-dose imatinib mesylate with or without peg-interferon and GM-CSF as frontline therapy for patients with chronic myeloid leukemia in early chronic phase. Blood 2005 (ASH annual meeting abstract); 106:1084a.

9

Molecular Targets Other Than *BCR-ABL*: How to Incorporate Them into the CML Therapy?

Junia V. Melo and David J. Barnes

Department of Haematology, Imperial College London, Hammersmith Hospital, London, U.K.

INTRODUCTION

The success of imatinib mesylate demonstrates the value of rational drug design based on detailed knowledge of a molecular target. However, the dangers of relying on sustained monotherapy against a single, precisely defined target are clearly illustrated by the substantial number of chronic myeloid leukemia (CML) patients who have now developed clinical resistance to imatinib. In this review, we will consider alternatives to Bcr-Abl tyrosine kinase inhibitors (TKI) and to immunotherapy in CML. Some of these targets are to be found in signaling pathways downstream of Bcr-Abl, such as the Ras-Raf-MAPK and PI-3K-Akt-mTOR pathways, which undergo abnormal and sustained signaling in *BCR-ABL* transformed cells. Other inhibitors act on targets, such as histone deacetylase and DNA methyltransferase, where no direct link with Bcr-Abl has been established. A minority of the inhibitors described in this review, including arsenic trioxide and perhaps, adaphostin, have no clearly defined target or exert their antileukemic effect via multiple mechanisms. In many, but not all, cases these compounds have demonstrated favorable interactions when combined with imatinib in the in vitro assays. For these agents, further to in vitro, in vivo and clinical studies are warranted, particularly where activity against imatinib resistant cells has been demonstrated.

HEAT-SHOCK PROTEIN 90 INHIBITORS

Heat-shock protein 90 (Hsp90) has recently emerged as an attractive molecular target for the therapy of CML. Hsp90 functions as a molecular chaperone which interacts with "client" proteins including Raf, Akt, FLT-3, and Bcr-Abl (1). Interaction with Hsp90 is essential for maintaining the client proteins in a stable and functional conformation and requires binding of adenosine triphosphate (ATP) to the hydrophobic N-terminal pocket of Hsp90. Benzoquinone ansamycins such as geldanamycin and its less toxic derivative, 17-allylamino-17-demethoxygeldanamycin (17-AAG) (both from the National Cancer Institute, Bethesda, Maryland, U.S.A.) bind to the ATP-binding pocket of Hsp90, thereby inhibiting its ability to function as a chaperone(2). The moment the interaction between Hsp90 and its client protein has been disrupted, another chaperone, heat-shock protein 70 (Hsp70), is recruited. Hsp70 has the opposite function to Hsp90 and the interaction of this chaperone with the client protein leading to its polyubiquitinylation and degradation by the 26S proteasome(1). In vitro treatment of CML cell lines with geldanamycin and 17-AAG leads to the down regulation of p210$^{Bcr-Abl}$ protein and induces cell death by apoptosis(3,4).

Geldanamycin and 17-AAG were also found to inhibit the growth of murine cell lines transformed with *BCR-ABL*, containing the Abl-kinase domain mutations T315I and E255K(5). A more potent inhibitory effect was noted for the cell lines expressing mutant *BCR-ABL* proteins than for cell lines bearing the wild-type protein (5). Unfortunately, monotherapy with 17-AAG may be less effective in patients who develop resistance to imatinib due to the selection of clones, which overexpress *BCR-ABL* [currently estimated to be 13% of imatinib-resistant patients (6)]. Radujkovic et al. (7) have recently reported cross resistance for *BCR-ABL* over-expressing imatinib-resistant CML cell lines. Combination therapy with imatinib and 17-AAG may benefit these patients, however, as the same group found that combining these drugs led to synergistic inhibition of growth and induction of apoptosis in the cross resistant cell lines. Curiously, in vitro treatment of the imatinib-sensitive counterparts of the resistant cell lines resulted in antagonistic or, at best, additive effects. Radujkovic et al. also showed that 17-AAG, additionally, targets the P-glycoprotein (Pgp) multidrug resistance pump and may therefore be inhibiting imatinib efflux. Overexpression of Pgp contributed to the imatinib-resistance of one of the cell lines studied, LAMA84-R and 17-AAG induced a profound inhibition of Pgp activity as assayed by Rhodamine-123 efflux (7). These findings remain to be confirmed in other CML cell lines and in primary cells from leukemia patients. The combination of 17-AAG with a cinnamic hydro-xyamic acid histone deacetylase inhibitor, LBH589, was found to induce synergistic apoptosis in a human CML cell line (1). This combination was also found to be effective at inducing of apoptosis in imatinib-resistant primary CML blast crisis (BC) cells and in a human cell line, which had been transformed with *BCR-ABL* containing the T315I mutation in its kinase domain (1). In addition, the combination of histone deacetylase inhibitors, suberanoylanilide hydroxamic acid (SAHA), and sodium butyrate with 17-AAG resulted in synergistic apoptosis and mitochondrial dysfunction in CML cell lines and CD34$^+$ cells, obtained from three CML patients (8). Clinical evaluation of 17-AAG is currently under way and a phase I trial involving 30 patients with advanced malignancies (all solid tumors) has been completed (9). This study established that a maximum dose of 450 mg/m^2/week was tolerable and phase II trials at this dose have been recommended (9).

ADAPHOSTIN: TYROSINE KINASE INHIBITOR OR NON-TYROSINE KINASE INHIBITOR?

Adaphostin (NSC 680410, National Cancer Institute, Bethesda, Maryland, U.S.A.) is the adamanyl ester of the tyrphostin, AG957 (10). Tyrphostins are a group of structurally diverse compounds that were synthesized and evaluated as potential inhibitors of tyrosine kinases. AG957 was identified as a non-ATP inhibitor of p210$^{Bcr-Abl}$ (11), which interfered with the binding of protein substrates to this tyrosine kinase. Several lines of evidence suggest that, currently, adaphostin should be considered as a "non-TKI" agent. Although AG957 has been reported as being a potent inhibitor of the tyrosine kinase activity of Bcr-Abl, adaphostin is less potent in this respect (10). Furthermore, although adaphostin induced rapid apoptosis in K562 cells, its effect upon tyrosine phosphorylation was gradual with detectable phosphorylated species persisting for at least six hours (12). In contrast, imatinib treatment of the same cell line abrogated phosphorylation within an hour but led to a much slower induction of apoptosis (12). Clearly, the cytotoxic action of adaphostin on CML cells is mediated via a mechanism distinct from that of imatinib. Significantly, adaphostin has also been reported to induce cell death in human cell lines that do not express Bcr-Abl including Jurkat (T-cell acute lymphoblastic leukemia cells), HL-60 (promyelocytic leukemia cells), and ML-1 (acute myeloid leukemia cells) (11). These findings indicate that the pro-apoptotic activity of adaphostin cannot be solely due to an effect upon Bcr-Abl. Curiously, adaphostin does not exhibit selectivity for murine cell lines transformed with *BCR-ABL*, but it does cause a selective inhibition in the growth of CML granulocyte colony forming units (CFU-G), relative to normal progenitors (12).

Several groups have reported that in vitro treatment of cells with adaphostin results in a rapid (within eight hours) down regulation of p210$^{Bcr-Abl}$ protein (10–13). In addition, adaphostin treatment leads to a rapid rise in intracellular reactive oxygen species (ROS) in both Bcr-Abl expressing and nonexpressing cells (11,13). Pretreatment of cells with antioxidants diminishes the cytoxicity of adaphostin but has no effect upon the down regulation of Bcr-Abl protein indicating that this phenomenon precedes or parallels the generation of ROS (11,13). The down regulation of Bcr-Abl protein by adaphostin was similarly unaffected by proteasome inhibitors and an inhibitor of protein translation, cycloheximide (11). Decreased levels of p210$^{Bcr-Abl}$ protein have also been reported for cells treated with AG957 (10,14) and this has been attributed to the drug, causing covalent crosslinks between Bcr-Abl and its substrate proteins, Grb2 and Shc (14). It has been suggested that the p210$^{Bcr-Abl}$ band is lost from immunoblots as Bcr-Abl is "shifted" to higher molecular weight complexes (14).

The mechanism underlying the apparent selectivity of adaphostin for primary CML cells remains elusive. It has been postulated that since Bcr-Abl overexpression leads to the production of ROS in haematopoietic cells (15), adaphostin may be inducing cytotoxicity in CML cells by further stimulating ROS, leading to intolerable oxidative stress (13). Regardless of its mode of action, adaphostin is considered a promising therapeutic agent in CML and may be of particular benefit to patients who develop resistance to imatinib. Imatinib-resistant cells do not exhibit cross resistance to adaphostin (12,13) and the combination of the two drugs induces greater cell death than when the two drugs are induced as single compounds (12). Recently, murine cell lines transfected with *BCR-ABL* containing Abl-kinase domain mutations, including the T315I mutation, were shown to be sensitive to adaphostin (13). Intriguingly, Ph$^+$ leukemia samples obtained from patients who had developed resistance to imatinib were found to be more sensitive to adaphostin than the samples obtained from patients who had never received imatinib (13). Synergistic induction of apoptosis by the combination of adaphostin and bortezomib has recently been reported in an in vitro study, involving murine cell lines transformed with *BCR-ABL*, containing Abl-kinase domain mutations (E255K, T315I, M351T) (16). All of the mutants were susceptible to this combination. At the time of writing, Spring 2006, adaphostin was still undergoing preclinical evaluation at the National Cancer Institute, Bethesda, Maryland, U.S.A. (13).

TARGETING PATHWAYS DOWNSTREAM OF BCR-ABL
Ras-Mitogen-Activated Protein Kinase Signaling
A wealth of biochemical and genetic evidence indicates that Ras-signaling has a key role in the leukemic transformation initiated by Bcr-Abl. Ras proteins are 21 kDa

guanine-nucleotide binding proteins (G-proteins) encoded by the H-, K-, and N-RAS genes (17). In normal, untransformed cells, *Ras* proteins function as molecular switches that cycle between an inactive and an active state, in response to whichever of the guanine nucleotides, guanosine diphosphate (GDP), or guanosine triphosphate (GTP), occupy their binding site. Inactive Ras contains GDP and becomes activated when this is exchanged for GTP. Activated Ras binds to Raf-1, a serine-threonine kinase, which initiates the mitogen-activated protein kinase (MAPK) cascade. MAPK signaling is mitogenic as the terminal kinases in this pathway activate transcription factors that promote the transcription of genes, involved in cell division.

In CML, oncogenic Ras-signaling is stimulated by Bcr-Abl via intermediate "adapter proteins." Autophosphorylation of the tyrosine 177 residue on Bcr-Abl creates a binding site for one of these adapter proteins, Grb2. The bound Grb2 then associates with another adapter molecule, the "son of sevenless" (SoS) protein to form a complex, which activates Ras by functioning as a guanine nucleotide exchange factor facilitating the exchange of GTP for GDP. In addition, Ras may be activated by two other known substrates of *BCR-ABL*, which function as adapter proteins, Shc and CrkL.

FARNESYL TRANSFERASE AND GERANYLGERANYL TRANSFERASE INHIBITORS

To function correctly, Ras must be anchored to the plasma membrane. This is achieved by a posttranslational modification of Ras, which is catalysed by the enzyme farnesyl transferase (FT). FT activity leads to the covalent attachment of a 15-carbon isoprenoid group to the C-terminus of Ras, which serves to "tether" the G-protein to the membrane. Prenylation is essential and unprenylated Ras is non functional. Rational drug design has yielded farnesyl transferase inhibitors (FTI), which interfere with the FT activity required for the prenylation of Ras (18). With regard to the treatment of CML, two FTIs in particular, tipifarnib (formerly R115777; Johnson & Johnson Pharmaceutical Research and Development, Titusville, New Jersey, U.S.A.) and lonafarnib (formerly SCH66336; Schering-Plough, Kenilworth, New Jersey, U.S.A.) have demonstrated potential as antileukemic agents.

Tipifarnib has been the subject of phase I (17) and phase II (19) clinical trials. The former was conducted in a cohort of 35 patients with acute and poor-risk leukemias (17). Included within this cohort were three CML-BC patients of whom one was Ph-negative. Tipifarnib was administered orally according to a dose-escalation scheme from 100 mg to 1200 mg twice daily for 21 days. Whereas the Ph-negative patient failed to respond to the treatment, the remaining two CML patients achieved partial hematological responses with reduced peripheral white blood cell counts, normalization of platelet counts, and decreased numbers of blasts in bone marrow and peripheral blood. In contrast to the Ph-negative patient, who died within six months, both of these individuals were alive 14 and 11 months after receiving tipifarnib. Although the surviving patients were both Ph-positive (with complex cytogenetic re-arrangements), the presence of the Ph chromosome, per se, is not predictive of a favorable response to tipifarnib since three other patients in this trial had Ph-positive adult acute lymphoblastic leukemia (ALL) and failed to achieve a hematological response. Reproducible inhibition of farnesyl transferase activity could be demonstrated by a twice-daily dose of 600 mg of tipifarnib. When a 1200 mg dose was introduced twice daily, central nervous system toxicity was observed and was considered to be dose limiting.

A phase II trial of tipifarnib involved 22 patients with CML, eight with myelofibrosis and ten with multiple myeloma (19). Tipifarnib was administered orally at 600 mg twice daily for four weeks, every six weeks. The results were somewhat disappointing as the drug was found to have only modest activity, inducing complete or partial hematological responses in seven (32%) of the CML patients. Minor cytogenetic responses were also achieved by four of these seven patients. Responses were not sustained and the median duration was only nine weeks. Of the seven CML patients who achieved a response, six were in chronic phase (CP) and one was in accelerated phase (AP). In contrast to the phase I trial, none of the six (27%) BC patients, who entered in this phase II trial, responded to tipifarnib. A correlation was noted between favorable responses to tipifarnib and a reduction in plasma levels of vascular endothelial growth factor (VEGF), a mediator of angiogenesis. This finding may indicate a role for VEGF in the pathogenesis or progression of CML, but further studies will be required to determine whether the antileukemic activity of tipifarnib is mediated via an inhibitory effect upon this cytokine (19).

Lonafarnib is the other FTI to show promise as an antileukemic agent. This compound has been shown to be a potent and selective inhibitor of the growth of primary cells from CML patients (18). In contrast, the growth of bone marrow cells from healthy individuals, as assessed in the same in vitro assay, was only modestly inhibited by lonafarnib at a dose that was ten-fold higher than that which completely inhibited the growth of the CML cells. Furthermore, lonafarnib demonstrated efficacy against Bcr-Abl-induced acute leukemia in a murine model of CML-BC (18). There were initial hopes that lonafarnib might prove useful for treating CML patients who had become refractory to treatment with imatinib. In an in vitro study, lonafarnib inhibited the proliferation of imatinib-resistant cell lines and reduced colony formation by primary cells obtained from patients, who were unresponsive to imatinib (20). However, the results of a pilot study into the efficacy of lonafarnib in CML patients, who were resistant or refractory to imatinib therapy have been discouraging (21). Of 13 patients (6 CP, 7 AP) who received an oral dose of 200 mg of lonafarnib twice daily, only two responded (21). Lonafarnib may still be therapeutically useful, however. A recent report has shown that lonafarnib is able to sensitize a rare population of Bcr-Abl-positive CD34$^+$ progenitors that remain "quiescent" and innately insensitive to imatinib (22). Treatment of this population with Ara-C alone or L294002 alone blocked their proliferation but did not kill them. Cotreatment with Ara-C, LY294002 or 17-AAG with imatinib enhanced the cytostatic effect of imatinib but did not prevent the surviving cells from growing again. Only the combination of lonafarnib and imatinib was effective in depleting this insensitive population (22).

Although tipifarnib and lonafarnib have shown potential as antileukemic agents, they suffer from a limitation common to all FTIs, which is that inhibition of farnesyl transferase does not ensure complete abrogation of Ras-signaling. This is because Ras may be prenylated, and hence anchored to the plasma membrane to assume a functional state, via an alternative pathway involving another enzyme, geranylgeranyl transferase-1 (GGT) (23). Consequently, therapeutic agents, which are capable of inhibiting both pathways, are being sought.

One such compound is zoledronate, a heterocyclic imidazole, which was developed as a third-generation bisphosphonate for the treatment of bone disorders. Zoledronate antagonizes the intracellular mevalonate pathway that generates geranylgeranyl pyrophosphate and farnesyl pyrophosphate, thus depleting cells of the substrates required for either farnesylation or geranylgeranylation of Ras. This compound has been shown to inhibit the growth of 2 human Ph^+ leukemia cell lines in vitro and to prolong the survival of non-obese diabetic/severe combined immunodeficient (NOD/SCID) mice that had been injected with the CML cell line, BV173 (23). In addition, a synergistic effect upon survival could be demonstrated in mice treated with both zoledronate and imatinib. This finding indicates that the combination of zoledronate and imatinib may be of value in the treatment of CML. We have recently shown that the combination of zoledronate and imatinib has additive to synergistic effects in in vitro assays, and that zoledronate effectively inhibits the growth of imatinib-resistant CML cell lines, including three mutations with Abl-kinase domain mutations (Y253F, E255K, and M351T) (24). Our findings are in contrast to those of Segawa et al. (25) who found that zoledronate or imatinib alone or in combination were ineffective in vitro against primary cells harboring the E255K and T315 mutations. There remains uncertainty about the bioavailability of zoledronate. Although doubts have been expressed as to whether effective serum concentrations of the drug can be achieved in vivo or not, these must be set against the high affinity of zoledronate for mineralized bone, which would, otherwise, tend to concentrate it in the bone marrow (23). It has been recommended that zoledronate should be evaluated for efficacy against Ph^+ leukemia in a phase I clinical trial (23).

MEK1/2 INHIBITORS

Downstream of Ras, Raf-1 activates the MAPK kinases, MEK1/2 (MAPK or ERK Kinase). MEK1/2 are dual specificity kinases, which in turn, activate Extracellular signal-Regulated Kinase 1/2 (ERK1/2). Several MEK1/2 inhibitors have been developed, including PD098059 (26), PD184352 (27) (Parke-Davis, Ann Arbor, Michigan, U.S.A.), and U0126 (28) (DuPont Merck, Wilmington, Delaware, U.S.A.). In vitro treatment of a CML cell line with PD098059 induced apoptosis (26) and PD184352, PD098059 or U0126, when combined with imatinib, caused synergistic induction of apoptosis in CML cell lines (27). Similarly, U0126 combined with imatinib was shown to significantly inhibit proliferation of CML $CD34^+$ progenitor cells (28). In addition, the combination of PD184352 and imatinib effectively induced cell death in an imatinib-resistant cell line, which overexpressed Bcr-Abl (27). Recently, a synergistic increase in mitochondrial damage, caspase activation, and apoptosis was demonstrated in CML cell lines and CML $CD34^+$ progenitors that were treated with the combinations of MEK1/2 inhibitors (PD184352 and U0126) and histone deacetylase inhibitors (suberanoylanilide hydroxamic acid and sodium butyrate) (29). At present, data on these compounds is limited to their activity in vitro. It remains to be seen whether MEK inhibitors will show efficacy in vivo. In addition, it should be borne in mind that MEK signaling is essential for normal cell physiology and that blocking these signals may result in unwanted toxic side-effects. These may limit the clinical usefulness of MEK inhibitors for the molecular therapy of CML.

PI-3 KINASE-AKT-mTOR SIGNALING

BCR-ABL activates phosphatidylinositol-3 (PI-3) kinase via a direct association with its 85 kDa regulatory subunit (30). Signaling via the PI-3 kinase is essential for the growth of CML, but not normal, progenitors (30). The PI-3 kinase inhibitors, wortmannin and LY294002 (Lilly, Indianapolis, Indiana, U.S.A.) have been shown to reproduce the selective antiproliferative effect of imatinib by inhibiting the clonogenic growth of CML progenitors but not that of normal progenitor cells (31). In addition, the combination of imatinib and wortmannin exerted a synergistic inhibitory effect upon the growth of CML cell lines (32). Imatinib combined with wortmannin or LY294002 was also effective in inhibiting colony formation by primary cells obtained from patients in CP or BC (32). The clinical usefulness of wortmannin, however, is severely limited by its instability in aqueous solution. LY294002 has superior stability but is less potent than wortmannin with an IC_{50} for PI-3 kinase, that has been reported as being 70-(33) to 300-fold (34) higher than that of wortmannin. Newer compounds, such as ZSTK474, offer the possibility of improved solubility and potencies to match that of wortmannin (33).

mTOR INHIBITORS

There is currently considerable interest in agents that antagonize the mammalian target of rapamycin (mTOR), a serine-threonine kinase downstream of PI-3 kinase, which is activated upon phosphorylation by Akt (35). As its name suggests, mTOR is specifically inhibited by the macrolide antibiotic rapamycin [Rapamune® (sirolimus); Wyeth Pharmaceuticals, Collegeville, Pennsylvania, U.S.A.]. Rapamycin binds to the immunophilin molecule, FKBP12, and the resulting complex inhibits mTOR (35). Recently, a derivative of rapamycin, RAD001 [Certican® (everolimus); Novartis Pharma, Basel, Switzerland], has been developed, which has superior oral bioavailability (36). The importance of mTOR as a potential target for molecular therapy in CML was first recognized by Ly et al. (35) who used an Akt phospho substrate specific antibody to detect substrates of serine/threonine kinases containing phosphorylation of serine or threonine residues within a consensus motif. By combining 2D-electrophoresis with a proteomics search, they identified two species that were constitutively phosphorylated in lysates of Bcr-Abl-expressing cell lines. These phosphorylated substrates were ribosomal protein S6 and the eukaryotic initiation factor 4E-binding protein-1 (4E-BP1). Experiments with rapamycin, LY294002 and imatinib indicated that both ribosomal protein S6 and 4E-BP1 were phosphorylated via the Bcr-Abl-PI-3K-Akt-mTOR pathway. In addition, these authors showed that another kinase, p70S6-kinase1 (p70S6K1) downstream of mTOR, was ultimately responsible for the phosphorylation of ribosomal protein S6. Abnormal and sustained activation of the PI-3K-Akt-mTOR pathway by Bcr-Abl is likely to result in altered translation of critical, although as yet unidentified, target genes, since ribosomal protein S6 and 4E-BP1 are both translational regulators. In this regard, a phenotype consisting of increased production of ROS has been identified with stimulation of the PI-3K-Akt-mTOR pathway in Bcr-Abl-transformed cells (37). It has been suggested that the increase in ROS is secondary to abnormally elevated glucose metabolism and an overactive mitochondrial electron transport chain (37).

Although Ly et al. (35) found that rapamycin alone had negligible effects upon the growth of a murine cell line transformed with Bcr-Abl (Ba/F3-Bcr-Abl), subsequent reports have suggested that this compound is effective at inhibiting the growth of Bcr-Abl-expressing cells. Hence, treatment with rapamycin alone has been shown to inhibit the growth of Ba/F3-Bcr-Abl (36,38) as well as Bcr-Abl-transformed B lymphoblasts (38) and primary CML cells (39), and to prolong the survival of Balb/C mice transplanted with bone marrow that had been retrovirally transduced with Bcr-Abl (38). The inhibitory effect of rapamycin on the in vitro growth of primary CML cells is due to induction of G1 cell cycle arrest and the induction of apoptosis (39). Down regulation of VEGF expression in cells treated with rapamycin has been reported by Mayerhofer et al. (39), but these authors discount the possibility that this is responsible for the compound's inhibitory effect on cell growth, since exogenously applied VEGF did not restore cell proliferation in rapamycin treated cells. Reduced levels of VEGF may still contribute to an antileukemic effect, however, and it is of note that treatment with the FTI tipifarnib is also associated with depletion of VEGF (19).

Disparate findings have been published regarding the effects of the combination of rapamycin with imatinib on imatinib resistant cells. This combination has been demonstrated to be effective at suppressing the growth of imatinib resistant murine cell lines in which the mechanism of resistance is overexpression of Bcr-Abl, but to have no effect upon the growth of murine cell lines with "strong" imatinib-resistance due to the T315I Abl-kinase domain mutation (35).

In contrast, rapamycin and imatinib have been shown to inhibit the growth of murine cell lines containing two mutations, which confer strong imatinib-resistance (T315I and E255K), but the levels of inhibition due to the combination were no better than those achieved with rapamycin alone (36). Synergism between rapamycin and imatinib could be demonstrated for a murine cell line containing a mutation, F317V, which is known to confer "weak" imatinib-resistance on cells (36). Similar findings were obtained with the combination of RAD001 and imatinib (36). These results are consistent with the notion that drug combinations with imatinib are more likely to exhibit synergistic activity if at least some effect can be achieved with imatinib alone (as is the case for mutations that confer weak imatinib resistance) (40). There are, however, reports of synergism between rapamycin and imatinib in cells containing the mutations responsible for strong imatinib resistance. Hence synergistic inhibition of growth has been described for murine lines containing the Y253F, E255K mutations (39), and T315I mutations (36). In the latter case, a "3-way" synergism involving rapamycin, imatinib and a MEK inhibitor, U0126, was also demonstrated (38). It is unclear why some groups report synergistic growth inhibition for the combination of imatinib and rapamycin in cell lines with strong imatinib resistance and others do not. Differences between the cellular models used are unlikely to be responsible since these studies were carried out using Bcr-Abl mutants expressed in the same murine cell line (BaF/3). Additional in vitro assays using a wider range of imatinib-resistant cell lines will be required to resolve this question.

Recently, signaling via the PI-3K-Akt-mTOR pathway has been implicated as a compensatory mechanism responsible for maintaining the viability of imatinib-naïve cells upon first exposure to imatinib (41). Treatment of the CML line LAMA84 with imatinib led to activation of PI-3K-Akt-mTOR signaling and phosphorylation of the down stream substrate p70S6K1. Clones of the treated cells grew in the presence of imatinib but they had not, at least initially, acquired "strong" imatinib-resistance via a Bcr-Abl dependent mechanism. Survival of the cells was attributed to "incipient" imatinib-resistance as a consequence of

PI-3K-Akt-mTOR signaling (41). Continued culture in imatinib led to the selection of subclones which had acquired "overt" resistance via overexpression of Bcr-Abl or through mutation of the Abl-kinase domain. Similar results were obtained with primary cells obtained from CML patients. Treatment of cells with rapamycin prevented activation of Akt by imatinib and retarded the development of imatinib resistance. It is unlikely that PI-3K-Akt-mTOR signaling contributes substantially to "overt" imatinib resistance, as only a minority of imatinib-resistant patients had evidence of activation of Akt or p70S6K1 (41). These findings would suggest that rapamycin treatment would mostly benefit imatinib-sensitive patients. Collectively, the in vitro studies with rapamycin and RAD001 suggest that these agents show promise as antileukemic compounds. Clinical trials to establish their efficacy in CML are now required. Treatment of one BC CML patient with rapamycin has been reported (39). Rapamycin was administered orally at 2 mg/daily for 17 consecutive days. The treatment resulted in reduced numbers of peripheral blood leukocytes and blasts as well as a decrease in Bcr-Abl transcript levels. Following discontinuation of rapamycin treatment on day 17, there was no increase in the number of blast cells during the following four weeks (39).

Although the results obtained, so far, from the in vitro studies of rapamycin combined with imatinib have been somewhat contradictory, the rationale for combining these agents with the aim of increasing their efficacy is impeccable. As outlined by Mohi et al. (38) the imatinib/rapamycin (or RAD001) combination is likely to prove worthwhile for several reasons. These include: both drugs have known mechanisms of action and are already used clinically (rapamycin being used for immunosuppression following organ transplantation), both are well tolerated at serum levels above those used in the in vitro studies, and the development path for two approved drugs is likely to be shorter than that for two novel agents. The last point holds out the promise of benefiting patients more rapidly than could otherwise be achieved (38).

HISTONE DEACETYLASE INHIBITORS

Histone deacetylases (HDAC) catalyse the deacetylation of lysine residues at the amino termini of core nucleosomal histones (42). This process is associated with chromatin relaxation and uncoiling, which permits the transcription of various genes including the key cyclin-dependent kinase inhibitor, p21 (42). By inhibiting HDAC, histone deacetylase inhibitors (HDI) cause hyperacetylation of histones. Hyperacetylation of histone H3 leads to transcriptional up regulation of p21, cell cycle arrest and apoptosis in tumor cells (42,43). The HDI acid SAHA induced p21 expression in one of the two CML cell lines and induced expression of p27, a key cell cycle regulator, in both of them (42). SAHA treatment was also associated with down regulation of p210$^{Bcr-Abl}$ protein. Combination treatment of CML cell lines with SAHA and imatinib resulted in a greater level of apoptosis than was achieved with either agent alone (42,44). This combination also produced synergistic induction of apoptosis in imatinib-resistant CML cell lines, which overexpressed Bcr-Abl (44). Ectopic expression of constitutively active MEK1/2 in a CML cell line attenuated apoptosis induced by the combination of SAHA and imatinib, suggesting that disruption of the Raf-MEK/ERK pathway by this drug combination may be involved in the synergistic antileukemia effect (44). In vitro treatment with SAHA alone of CD34$^+$ cells, obtained from a patient who had progressed to BC while receiving imatinib, was sufficient to down regulate Bcr-Abl protein levels and to induce apoptosis (42). Another HDI, LAQ824 (Novartis Pharma, Basel, Switzerland), a cinnamyl hydroxamic acid analogue, was found to induce the expression of p21 and p27 in CML BC cells and to induce apoptosis (43). Co-treatment of CML BC cells with LAQ824 and imatinib increased imatinib-induced apoptosis. In addition, LAQ824 induced acetylation of Hsp90, inhibiting its association with p210$^{Bcr-Abl}$, and leading to degradation of the oncoprotein (43). The latter finding provided the rationale for studying the effect of the combination of another HDI, LBH589, with the Hsp90 antagonist, 17-AAG (1). This combination was found to induce synergistic apoptosis in a CML cell line, and to effectively induce apoptosis in a human cell line engineered to express Bcr-Abl containing the T315I Abl-kinase domain mutation (1). Similar findings were obtained when CML cell lines were subjected to co-treatment with 17-AAG and either of the HDIs SAHA and sodium butyrate (8). These combinations caused synergistic apoptosis and mitochondrial dysfunction both in the cell lines and in CD34$^+$ cells taken from three CML patients (8). Recently, the HDI valproate, which is commonly administered as a treatment for epilepsy, was found to enhance imatinib-induced growth arrest and apoptosis in CML cell lines when combined with this TKI (45). In addition, valproate sensitized imatinib-resistant CML cell lines and imatinib-resistant primary mononuclear cells to imatinib and restored its cytotoxic effect. Treatment with valproate was associated with down regulation of the anti-apoptotic gene product Bcl-2. This finding challenges the accepted model, which the HDI induce up regulation of genes. Whereas other HDI are associated with toxic side effects, valproate is currently in therapeutic use. It has been suggested that valproate could easily be combined with imatinib (45).

PROTEASOME INHIBITORS

Proteasome inhibitors target the catalytic 20S core of the proteasome thereby suppressing the proteasomal degradation of numerous cellular proteins (46). For reasons that are only partly understood, proteasome inhibitors induce apoptosis in tumor cells but are relatively sparing in normal cells. Consequently, these compounds have shown potential as antineoplastic agents. Inhibition of transcription activated by nuclear factor κB (NF-κB) has been implicated as the mechanism that is ultimately responsible for the antitumor effect of proteasome inhibitors. In particular, these compounds are thought to impair the translocation of NF-κB into the nucleus by preventing the proteasomal degradation of its endogenous inhibitor, P-IκB (47). In CML, the proteasome inhibitor that has been studied most intensively is the dipepityl boronic acid bortezomib (Velcade®, PS-341; Millenium Pharmaceuticals, Cambridge, Massachusetts, U.S.A.) (46–48). Bortezomib inhibited the growth of imatinib-sensitive and resistant CML cell lines in a dose-dependent manner (47). In vitro, treatment with bortezomib was also associated with an accumulation of cells in the G2/M phase of the cell cycle, activation of caspase 3, and the induction of apoptosis. Reduced NF-κB binding to DNA was observed, but this was only transient and was not correlated with the induction of apoptosis (47). However, apoptotic cell death was accompanied by down regulation of p210$^{Bcr-Abl}$ protein (47). Although, sequential exposure of CML cell lines to low doses of bortezomib followed by imatinib resulted in additive effects upon growth inhibition, the simultaneous treatment of imatinib-sensitive CML cell lines with these drugs produced an antagonistic interaction. Consequently, caution will need to be exercised in the design of any possible future clinical trials involving the combination of bortezomib with imatinib (47). Synergism between bortezomib and the histone deacetylase inhibitor SAHA (46) and between bortezomib and flavopiridol (48) have been reported in the in vitro studies of growth inhibition of CML cell lines. In addition, the former combination led to an increased apoptosis, relative to the level obtained for either drug alone, in an imatinib-resistant CML cell line, in which Bcr-Abl was overexpressed, or in $CD34^+$ cells from a patient with imatinib-resistant disease (46). The latter combination exhibited additivity in a Bcr-Abl-overexpressing imatinib-resistant CML line and in a second resistant CML line with reduced expression of Bcr-Abl but increased expression and activation of the Lyn and Hck kinases (48). The synergism between adaphostin and bortezomib in murine cell lines transfected with mutant forms of Bcr-Abl has been described previously (16). These findings suggest that further preclinical and clinical trials are required to identify drugs that exhibit additivity or synergism with botezomib (or another suitable proteasome inhibitor) and, just as importantly, to identify combinations, which may result in antagonism.

CYCLIN-DEPENDENT KINASE INHIBITORS

Multiple cyclin-dependent kinases (CDKs) including, CDK1, CDK2, CDK4/6, and CDK7, are targeted by the semi-synthetic flavone, flavopiridol (L86–8275, HMR 1275; National Cancer Institute, Bethesda, Maryland, U.S.A.) (49). Co-treatment with imatinib and flavopiridol led to increased mitochondrial damage, activation of caspases and apoptosis in CML cell lines but not in leukemia cell lines that did not express Bcr-Abl (49). In addition, this drug combination effectively induced apoptosis in an imatinib-resistant CML cell line that overexpressed Bcr-Abl (49). As mentioned earlier, synergistic induction of apoptosis has been reported for the combination of flavopiridol and the proteasome inhibitor, bortezomib, in imatinib-sensitive and resistant CML cell lines (48). Unlike some of the other therapeutic agents previously discussed, flavopiridol has only recently been recognized as a potential treatment for CML. A phase I trial to identify appropriate dose combinations of imatinib and flavopiridol was conducted in 2005 in 21 patients with Bcr-Abl-positive hematologic malignancies (50). This combination was found to be tolerable and was responsible for four objective responses, including two complete hematologic remissions (50). Further clinical trials will be required to establish the efficacy of drug combinations containing flavopiridol.

DNA-METHYLTRANSFERASE INHIBITORS

Epigenetic changes are a characteristic feature of human leukemias and many gene promoters exhibit abnormally high methylation (51). Methylation of promoter sequences contributes to the malignant phenotype of transformed cells by silencing genes that are essential for differentiation and apoptosis. Consequently, there is much interest in DNA hypomethylating agents, which inhibit the enzymes that catalyse this aberrant methylation. Docitabine (5-aza-2'-deoxycytidine; SuperGen, Dublin, California, U.S.A.) is a DNA hypomethylating agent that shows promise as a therapeutic agent for the treatment of CML (51). This compound integrates into DNA and forms irreversible covalent bonds with DNA-methyltransferase (Mtase) at cytosine residues targeted for methylation. DNA synthesis stalls at these covalently modified sites and the DNA-Mtase complexes are eventually degraded. Loss of the Mtase-DNA complexes is associated with depletion of

Mtase levels and, when renewed DNA synthesis occurs; the newly synthesized DNA is hypomethylated. Promoters silenced by methylation become reactivated and their genes are expressed (51).

In a study of 130 CML patients who received decitabine, objective responses were achieved by 28% of patients in BC, 55% in AP and 63% in CP (52). Decitabine was administered at $100 \, \text{mg/m}^2$ over six hours every 12 hours for five days ($1,000 \, \text{mg/m}^2$ per course) in the first 13 patients, at $75 \, \text{mg/m}^2$ in the subsequent 33 patients, and at $50 \, \text{mg/m}^2$ in the remaining 84 patients. These doses were associated with severe myelosuppression that was delayed, prolonged, and dose-dependent. Decitabine is likely to be more efficacious when administered at lower doses and for longer periods of time as evidenced by the results of a recent phase I trial in relapsed or refractory leukemias (51). In this study, decitabine was given to 50 patients of whom 44 had acute myeloid leukemia/myelodysplasia, five had CML (one CP, one AP, three BC), and one had acute lymphocytic leukemia. Low dose prolonged exposure schedules of decitabine were used so that patients received the drug at 5, 10, 15, or $20 \, \text{mg/m}^2$ intravenously over one hour daily, five days a week, for two consecutive weeks. Of the five CML patients, two (40%) achieved complete responses and two (40%) partial responses. Overall, the best responses were obtained with the dose of $15 \, \text{mg/m}^2$ for ten days (11 of 17, 65%), whereas fewer responses were achieved when the dose was escalated or prolonged (2 of 19, 11%). Significantly, the two CML patients who achieved complete responses were both treated with $15 \, \text{mg/m}^2$ decitabine for ten days. It has been postulated that decitabine may exert dual effects depending upon the dose (51). At high doses, treated cells undergo apoptosis and cell death triggered by the presence of DNA adducts and stalled replication forks. In contrast, at lower doses cells survive, but with an altered expression profile that favors differentiation and reduced proliferation. Regardless, of the mechanism of action, it is likely that the future of decitabine therapy in CML lies in low dose prolonged exposure regimens. Decitabine may prove useful when combined with imatinib, as an in vitro study revealed that this combination had additive to synergistic growth inhibitory effects upon imatinib-resistant Bcr-Abl-expressing cell lines (40). Although this combination inhibited the growth of cells containing mutant forms of Bcr-Abl with the M351T and Y253F Abl-kinase domain mutations, imatinib and decitabine were found to be less potent than decitabine, by itself, at inhibiting the growth of cells with the T315I mutant.

ARSENIC TRIOXIDE

Arsenic compounds are some of the oldest treatments for leukemia. Potassium arsenite, Fowler's solution, was used to treat leukemia patients in the 19th and early 20th centuries and some impressive clinical responses were achieved (53). Arsenic trioxide (As_2O_3, Trisenox®; Cell Therapeutics, Inc., Seattle, Washington, U.S.A.) has been demonstrated to induce apoptosis in Bcr-Abl-positive but not negative lymphoid cell lines and to reduce the proliferation of CML blasts but not of peripheral $CD34^+$ progenitors (53). Apoptosis induced in CML cell lines was found to be associated with the cytosolic accumulation of cytochrome c and pre-apoptotic mitochondrial events, such as the loss of inner membrane potential and an increase in ROS (54). Recently it has been shown that As_2O_3 induced apoptosis occurs via the endoplasmic reticulum stress mediated pathway of cell apoptosis (55). It has also been reported that As_2O_3 treatment of CML cell lines inhibits the translation of *BCR-ABL* mRNA leading to attenuation of cellular levels of the onco-protein (56). In the in vitro studies, the combination of As_2O_3 with imatinib was found to induce additive to synergistic inhibition of the growth of Bcr-Abl-expres-sing cell lines (57), and to induce cell death in imatinib-resistant cell lines, which overexpressed Bcr-Abl or had the M351T or Y253F, but not the T315I, Abl-kinase domain mutations (40). This latter finding suggests that the combination of imatinib with As_2O_3 may only be of clinical benefit if the mechanism of imatinib-resistance is still susceptible to dose escalation of imatinib-monotherapy (40). Hence, there is renewed interest in the potential of arsenic compounds for the treatment of CML but in a novel context of agents that can be combined with other drugs to yield synergistic effects.

CONCLUSION

In reviewing the available treatment options based on nonimmunological and non-TKI targets, it becomes apparent that viable therapies involving these targets are likely to emerge, if at all, more rapidly in some cases than others. This is especially true of therapeutic agents that have already been approved for use in humans (but for other purposes) such as rapamycin, zoledronate, and valproate. These drugs have already been the subject of clinical trials and any toxic effects have already been identified. However, some of the other inhibitors described in this review, such as 17-AAG and adaphostin, are currently subjected to preclinical or clinical evaluation and ultimately may prove to be equally efficacious as, or more so, than the licensed drugs. Efforts to identify synergistic drug combinations are obviously essential and it is likely that the in vitro studies, involving novel combi-nations, will continue to play an important part in CML research.

REFERENCES

1. George P, Bali P, Annavarapu S, et al. Combination of the histone deacetylase inhibitor LBH589 and the hsp90 inhibitor 17-AAG is highly active against human CML-BC cells and AML cells with activating mutation of FLT-3. Blood 2005; 105:1768–1776.
2. Schulte TW, Neckers LM. The benzoquinone ansamycin 17-allylamino-17-demethoxy-geldanamycin binds to HSP90 and shares important biologic activities with geldanamy-cin. Cancer Chemother Pharmacol 1998; 42:273–279.
3. Nimmanapalli R, O'Bryan E, Bhalla K. Geldanamycin and its analogue 17-allylamino-17-demethoxygeldanamycin lowers Bcr-Abl levels and induces apoptosis and differen-tiation of Bcr- Abl-positive human leukemic blasts. Cancer Res 2001; 61:1799–1804.
4. Nimmanapalli R, O'Bryan E, Huang M, et al. Molecular Characterization and Sensitivity of STI-571 (Imatinib Mesylate, Gleevec)-resistant, Bcr-Abl-positive, Human Acute Leu-kemia Cells to SRC Kinase Inhibitor PD180970 and 17-Allylamino-17- demethoxygelda-namycin. Cancer Res 2002; 62:5761–5769.
5. Gorre ME, Ellwood-Yen K, Chiosis G, Rosen N, Sawyers CL. *BCR-ABL* point mutants isolated from patients with imatinib mesylate- resistant chronic myeloid leukemia remain sensitive to inhibitors of the *BCR-ABL* chaperone heat shock protein 90. Blood 2002; 100:3041–3044.
6. Hochhaus A, Kreil S, Corbin AS, et al. Molecular and chromosomal mechanisms of resistance to imatinib (STI571) therapy. Leukemia 2002; 16:2190–2196.
7. Radujkovic A, Schad M, Topaly J, et al. Synergistic activity of imatinib and 17-AAG in imatinib-resistant CML cells overexpressing *BCR-ABL* - Inhibition of P-glycoprotein function by 17-AAG. Leukemia 2005; 19:1198–1206.
8. Rahmani M, Reese E, Dai Y, et al. Cotreatment with suberanoylanilide hydroxamic acid and 17-allylamino 17-demethoxygeldanamycin synergistically induces apoptosis in

Bcr-Abl+ Cells sensitive and resistant to STI571 (imatinib mesylate) in association with down-regulation of Bcr-Abl, abrogation of signal transducer and activator of transcription 5 activity, and Bax conformational change. Mol Pharmacol 2005; 67:1166–1176.

9. Banerji U, O'Donnell A, Scurr M, et al. Phase I pharmacokinetic and pharmacodynamic study of 17-allylamino, 17-demethoxygeldanamycin in patients with advanced malignancies. J Clin Oncol 2005; 23:4152–4161.

10. Svingen PA, Tefferi A, Kottke TJ, et al. Effects of the bcr/abl kinase inhibitors AG957 and NSC 680410 on chronic myelogenous leukemia cells in vitro. Clin Cancer Res 2000; 6:237–249.

11. Chandra J, Hackbarth J, Le S, et al. Involvement of reactive oxygen species in adaphostin-induced cytotoxicity in human leukemia cells. Blood 2003; 102:4512–4519.

12. Mow BM, Chandra J, Svingen PA, et al. Effects of the Bcr/abl kinase inhibitors STI571 and adaphostin (NSC 680410) on chronic myelogenous leukemia cells in vitro. Blood 2002; 99:664–671.

13. Chandra J, Tracy J, Loegering D, et al. Adaphostin-induced oxidative stress overcomes BCR/ABL mutation-dependent and -independent imatinib resistance. Blood 2006; 107:2501–2506.

14. Kaur G, Sausville EA. Altered physical state of p210bcr-abl in tyrphostin AG957-treated K562 cells. Anticancer Drugs 1996; 7:815–824.

15. Sattler M, Verma S, Shrikhande G, et al. The BCR/ABL tyrosine kinase induces production of reactive oxygen species in hematopoietic cells. J Biol Chem 2000; 275:24273–24278.

16. Dasmahapatra G, Nguyen TK, Dent P, Grant S. Adaphostin and bortezomib induce oxidative injury and apoptosis in imatinib mesylate-resistant hematopoietic cells expressing mutant forms of Bcr/Abl. Leuk Res 2006.

17. Karp JE, Lancet JE, Kaufmann SH, et al. Clinical and biologic activity of the farnesyltransferase inhibitor R115777 in adults with refractory and relapsed acute leukemias: a phase 1 clinical-laboratory correlative trial. Blood 2001; 97:3361–3369.

18. Peters DG, Hoover RR, Gerlach MJ, et al. Activity of the farnesyl protein transferase inhibitor SCH66336 against BCR/ABL-induced murine leukemia and primary cells from patients with chronic myeloid leukemia. Blood 2001; 97:1404–1412.

19. Cortes J, AlBitar M, Thomas D, et al. Efficacy of the farnesyl transferase inhibitor R115777 in chronic myeloid leukemia and other hematologic malignancies. Blood 2003; 101:1692–1697.

20. Hoover RR, Mahon FX, Melo JV, Daley GQ. Overcoming STI571 resistance with the farnesyl transferase inhibitor SCH66336. Blood 2002; 100:1068–1071.

21. Borthakur G, Kantarjian H, Daley G, et al. Pilot study of lonafarnib, a farnesyl transferase inhibitor, in patients with chronic myeloid leukemia in the chronic or accelerated phase that is resistant or refractory to imatinib therapy. Cancer 2006; 106:346–352.

22. Jorgensen HG, Allan EK, Graham SM, et al. Lonafarnib reduces the resistance of primitive quiescent CML cells to imatinib mesylate in vitro. Leukemia. 2005; 19:1184–1191.

23. Kuroda J, Kimura S, Segawa H, et al. The third-generation bisphosphonate zoledronate synergistically augments the anti-Ph+ leukemia activity of imatinib mesylate. Blood 2003; 102:2229–2235.

24. Chuah C, Barnes DJ, Kwok M, et al. Zoledronate inhibits proliferation and induces apoptosis of imatinib-resistant chronic myeloid leukaemia cells. Leukemia 2005; 19:1896–1904.

25. Segawa H, Kimura S, Kuroda J, et al. Zoledronate synergises with imatinib mesylate to inhibit Ph primary leukaemic cell growth. Br J Haematol 2005; 130:558–560.

26. Kang CD, Yoo SD, Hwang BW, et al. The inhibition of ERK/MAPK not the activation of JNK/SAPK is primarily required to induce apoptosis in chronic myelogenous leukemic K562 cells. Leuk Res 2000; 24:527–534.

27. Yu C, Krystal G, Varticovksi L, et al. Pharmacologic mitogen-activated protein/extracellular signal-regulated kinase kinase/mitogen-activated protein kinase inhibitors interact synergistically with STI571 to induce apoptosis in Bcr/Abl-expressing human leukemia cells. Cancer Res 2002; 62:188–199.

28. Chu S, Holtz M, Gupta M, Bhatia R. *BCR/ABL* kinase inhibition by imatinib mesylate enhances MAP kinase activity in chronic myelogenous leukemia CD34+ cells. Blood 2004; 103:3167–3174.

29. Yu C, Dasmahapatra G, Dent P, Grant S. Synergistic interactions between MEK1/2 and histone deacetylase inhibitors in *BCR/ABL*+ human leukemia cells. Leukemia 2005; 19:1579–1589.

30. Skorski T, Kanakaraj P, Nieborowska-Skorska M, et al. Phosphatidylinositol-3 kinase activity is regulated by *BCR/ABL* and is required for the growth of Philadelphia chromosome-positive cells. Blood 1995; 86:726–736.

31. Marley SB, Lewis JL, Schneider H, Rudd CE, Gordon MY. Phosphatidylinositol-3 kinase inhibitors reproduce the selective antiproliferative effects of imatinib on chronic myeloid leukaemia progenitor cells. Br J Haematol 2004; 125:500–511.

32. Klejman A, Rushen L, Morrione A, Slupianek A, Skorski T. Phosphatidylinositol-3 kinase inhibitors enhance the anti-leukemia effect of STI571. Oncogene 2002; 21: 5868–5876.

33. Yaguchi S, Fukui Y, Koshimizu I, et al. Antitumor activity of ZSTK474, a new phosphatidylinositol 3-kinase inhibitor. J Natl Cancer Inst 2006; 98:545–556.

34. Walker EH, Pacold ME, Perisic O, et al. Structural determinants of phosphoinositide 3-kinase inhibition by wortmannin, LY294002, quercetin, myricetin, and staurosporine. Mol Cell 2000; 6:909–919.

35. Ly C, Arechiga AF, Melo JV, Walsh CM, Ong ST. Bcr-Abl kinase modulates the translation regulators ribosomal protein S6 and 4E-BP1 in chronic myelogenous leukemia cells via the mammalian target of rapamycin. Cancer Res 2003; 63:5716–5722.

36. Dengler J, von Bubnoff N, Decker T, Peschel C, Duyster J. Combination of imatinib with rapamycin or RAD001 acts synergistically only in Bcr-Abl-positive cells with moderate resistance to imatinib. Leukemia 2005; 19:1835–1838.

37. Kim JH, Chu SC, Gramlich JL, et al. Activation of the PI3K/mTOR pathway by *BCR-ABL* contributes to increased production of reactive oxygen species. Blood 2005; 105:1717–1723.

38. Mohi MG, Boulton C, Gu TL, et al. Combination of rapamycin and protein tyrosine kinase (PTK) inhibitors for the treatment of leukemias caused by oncogenic PTKs. Proc Natl Acad Sci USA 2004; 101:3130–3135.

39. Mayerhofer M, Aichberger KJ, Florian S, et al. Identification of mTOR as a novel bifunctional target in chronic myeloid leukemia: dissection of growth-inhibitory and VEGF-suppressive effects of rapamycin in leukemic cells. FASEB J 2005; 19:960–962.

40. La Rosee P, Johnson K, Corbin AS, et al. In vitro efficacy of combined treatment depends on the underlying mechanism of resistance in imatinib-resistant Bcr-Abl-positive cell lines. Blood 2004; 103:208–215.

41. Burchert A, Wang Y, Cai D, et al. Compensatory PI3-kinase/Akt/mTor activation regulates imatinib resistance development. Leukemia 2005; 19:1774–1782.

42. Nimmanapalli R, Fuino L, Stobaugh C, Richon V, Bhalla K. Cotreatment with the histone deacetylase inhibitor suberoylanilide hydroxamic acid (SAHA) enhances imatinib-induced apoptosis of Bcr-Abl-positive human acute leukemia cells. Blood 2003; 101:3236–3239.

43. Nimmanapalli R, Fuino L, Bali P, et al. Histone deacetylase inhibitor LAQ824 both lowers expression and promotes proteasomal degradation of Bcr-Abl and induces apoptosis of imatinib mesylate-sensitive or -refractory chronic myelogenous leukemia-blast crisis cells. Cancer Res 2003; 63:5126–5135.

44. Yu C, Rahmani M, Almenara J, et al. Histone deacetylase inhibitors promote STI571-mediated apoptosis in STI571-sensitive and -resistant Bcr/Abl+ human myeloid leukemia cells. Cancer Res 2003; 63:2118–2126.

45. Morotti A, Cilloni D, Messa F, et al. Valproate enhances imatinib-induced growth arrest and apoptosis in chronic myeloid leukemia cells. Cancer 2006; 106:1188–1196.

46. Yu C, Rahmani M, Conrad D, et al. The proteasome inhibitor bortezomib interacts synergistically with histone deacetylase inhibitors to induce apoptosis in Bcr/Abl+ cells sensitive and resistant to STI571. Blood 2003; 102:3765–3774.

47. Gatto S, Scappini B, Pham L, et al. The proteasome inhibitor PS-341 inhibits growth and induces apoptosis in Bcr/Abl-positive cell lines sensitive and resistant to imatinib mesylate. Haematologica 2003; 88:853–863.

48. Dai Y, Rahmani M, Pei XY, Dent P, Grant S. Bortezomib and flavopiridol interact synergistically to induce apoptosis in chronic myeloid leukemia cells resistant to imatinib mesylate through both Bcr/Abl-dependent and -independent mechanisms. Blood 2004; 104:509–518.

49. Yu C, Krystal G, Dent P, Grant S. Flavopiridol potentiates STI571-induced mitochondrial damage and apoptosis in *BCR-ABL*-positive human leukemia cells. Clin Cancer Res 2002; 8:2976–2984.

50. Grant S, Karp JE, Koc ON, et al. Phase I Study of Flavopiridol in Combination with Imatinib Mesylate (STI571, Gleevec) in Bcr/Abl+ Hematological Malignancies [abstract]. Blood 2005; 106:1102.

51. Issa JP, Garcia-Manero G, Giles FJ, et al. Phase 1 study of low-dose prolonged exposure schedules of the hypomethylating agent 5-aza-2′-deoxycytidine (decitabine) in hematopoietic malignancies. Blood 2004; 103:1635–1640.

52. Kantarjian HM, O'Brien S, Cortes J, et al. Results of decitabine (5-aza-2′deoxycytidine) therapy in 130 patients with chronic myelogenous leukemia. Cancer 2003; 98:522–528.

53. Puccetti E, Guller S, Orleth A, et al. *BCR-ABL* mediates arsenic trioxide-induced apoptosis independently of its aberrant kinase activity. Cancer Res 2000; 60:3409–3413.

54. Perkins C, Kim CN, Fang G, Bhalla KN. Arsenic induces apoptosis of multidrug-resistant human myeloid leukemia cells that express Bcr-Abl or overexpress MDR, MRP, Bcl-2, or Bcl-x(L). Blood 2000; 95:1014–1022.

55. Du Y, Wang K, Fang H, et al. Coordination of intrinsic, extrinsic, and endoplasmic reticulum-mediated apoptosis by imatinib mesylate combined with arsenic trioxide in chronic myeloid leukemia. Blood 2006; 107:1582–1590.

56. Nimmanapalli R, Bali P, O'Bryan E, et al. Arsenic trioxide inhibits translation of mRNA of bcr-abl, resulting in attenuation of Bcr-Abl levels and apoptosis of human leukemia cells. Cancer Res. 2003; 63:7950–7958.

57. La Rosee P, Shen L, Stoffregen EP, Deininger M, Druker BJ. No correlation between the proliferative status of Bcr-Abl positive cell lines and the proapoptotic activity of imatinib mesylate (Gleevec/Glivec). Hematol J 2003; 4:413–419.

10

Blastic Transformation of Chronic Myelogenous Leukemia: Does *BCR-ABL* Orchestrate Disease Progression?

Bruno Calabretta

Department of Microbiology and Immunology, Kimmel Cancer Center,
Thomas Jefferson Medical College, Philadelphia, Pennsylvania, U.S.A.

Danilo Perrotti

Human Cancer Genetics Program, Department of Molecular Virology,
Immunology and Medical Genetics and the Comprehensive Cancer Center,
The Ohio State University, Columbus, Ohio, U.S.A.

INTRODUCTION

Blast crisis is the terminal phase of chronic myeloid leukemia (CML), a clonal myeloproliferative disorder of the pluripotent hematopoietic stem cell, which typically evolves in three distinct clinical stages: chronic phase, accelerated phase, and blast crisis (reviewed in refs. 1,2). Blast crisis lasts only a few months and is characterized by the rapid expansion of myeloid or lymphoid differentiation-arrested blast cells (1,2). CML is consistently associated with an acquired genetic abnormality, the Philadelphia chromosome (Ph[1]), a shortened chromosome 22 resulting from a reciprocal translocation of the long arms of chromosomes 9 and 22 (1,2). This translocation generates the *BCR-ABL* fusion gene, which is translated in the p210$^{BCR-ABL}$ oncoprotein of almost all CML patients (1,2).

Expression of p210$^{BCR-ABL}$ is necessary and sufficient for malignant transformation, as demonstrated by in vitro assays and leukemogenesis in mice (3,4). Transition to blast crisis is the unavoidable outcome of CML, except in a cohort of patients receiving allogeneic bone marrow transplantation early in the chronic phase (5). The development of the *BCR-ABL* tyrosine kinase inhibitor imatinib mesylate (Gleevec™; formerly STI571) as the treatment of choice for chronic phase CML and its remarkable therapeutic effects suggests that blast crisis transition will be postponed for several years in a majority of CML patients (6). However, the persistence of *BCR-ABL* transcripts in a cohort of patients with complete cytogenetic response (7) and the resistance of the primitive CML stem cell to imatinib treatment (8) raises the possibility that treatment with imatinib alone might delay but not prevent disease progression. Furthermore, most of the CML patients in the accelerated and blastic phases of the disease are either refractory or develop resistance to imatinib monotherapy. In these patients with CML in blast crisis, imatinib resistance often depends on reactivation of *BCR-ABL* tyrosine kinase activity via mechanisms involving *BCR-ABL* overexpression, gene amplification, or mutations that suppress imatinib-mediated kinase inhibition (i.e., E255V and G250E) or disrupt imatinib binding (i.e., T315I) (9,10). Thus, development of imatinib resistance appears to predispose to blastic transformation. Although new phase 1 clinical trials with the dual Src-Abl inhibitor dasatinib (BMS-354825) and the selective Abl inhibitor nilotinib (AMN107) show encouraging results (11), as they suppress the activity of most *BCR-ABL* mutants (except T315I) (11), in vitro evidence suggests that resistance to these new compounds may develop through mechanisms involving the selection and expansion of *BCR-ABL*-positive cell clones carrying the T315I *BCR-ABL* mutant (12). Additionally, dasatinib, like imatinib, is not effective in killing the most primitive quiescent CML cells (8) and, therefore, it may also be ineffective in preventing disease progression.

The mechanisms responsible for transition of CML chronic phase to blast crisis remain poorly understood, although a reasonable assumption is that the unrestrained activity of *BCR-ABL* in hematopoietic stem/progenitor cells is the primary determinant of disease progression. No causal relationship has been demonstrated yet between *BCR-ABL* expression that specifically increases during disease progression in hematopoietic stem cells and committed myeloid progenitors (13–15), and the secondary genetic changes of CML BC. However, a plausible model of disease progression predicts that increased *BCR-ABL* expression promotes the secondary molecular and chromosomal changes essential for the expansion of cell clones with increasingly malignant characteristics, and remains crucial for the malignant phenotype even in advanced stages of the disease (Fig. 1).

According to this model, CML blast crisis would be expected to occur only in patients with an imatinib-resistant disease or in those developing resistance during treatment. Indeed, a recent study from the GIMEMA Working Party on CML reported that the early detection of *BCR-ABL* mutations in CML chronic phase

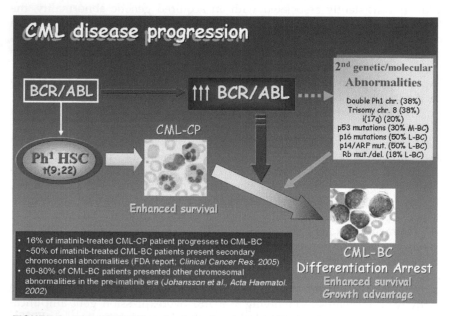

FIGURE 1 Does *BCR-ABL* orchestrate chronic myeloid leukemia disease progression? Increased expression of *BCR-ABL* may directly promote disease progression by influencing expression and function of important regulators of proliferation, survival and differentiation of malignant hematopoietic progenitors and also by enhancing genomic instability that, in turn, leads to emergence of secondary genetic and molecular abnormalities. *Abbreviations*: CML-CP, chronic myeloid leukemia-chronic phase; CML-BC, chronic myeloid leukemia-blastic phase.

patients is associated with a greater likelihood of disease progression (16). Interestingly, a direct correlation also seems to exist between levels of *BCR-ABL* and development of imatinib resistance (14,17). There is no evidence yet that imatinib-resistant patients have a clinically distinct disease; however, imatinib-resistant CML blast crisis patients may present distinct genetic abnormalities, the appearance of which could be influenced by the duration of *BCR-ABL*-dependent signals. Thus, the biology of CML blast crisis in the preimatinib and in the imatinib eras may be different. With this in mind, we will illustrate the molecular mechanisms underlying transition to CML blast crisis according to a model of disease progression in which (*i*) *BCR-ABL* activity is necessary for the accumulation of secondary genetic abnormalities and/or changes in gene expression; and (*ii*) such secondary events directly or indirectly promote differentiation arrest, the distinctive feature of CML blast crisis.

THE *BCR-ABL* SIGNALOSOME

In hematopoietic CML cells carrying the Ph[1] chromosome, the *BCR-ABL* fusion gene encodes p210$^{BCR-ABL}$, an oncoprotein which, unlike the normal p145 c-Abl, has constitutive tyrosine kinase activity and is predominantly localized in the cytoplasm (18). The tyrosine kinase activity is essential for cell transformation, and the cytoplasmic localization of *BCR-ABL* allows the assembly of phosphorylated substrates in multiprotein complexes that transmit mitogenic and antiapoptotic signals (18).

Ectopic expression of p210$^{BCR-ABL}$ results in growth factor independence and transformation of immortal hematopoietic cell lines (refer Refs. 1,3 and the references therein). Transplantation of *BCR-ABL*-transduced hematopoietic stem cells or transgenic expression of p210$^{BCR-ABL}$ induces leukemia and myeloproliferative disorders indicating a direct, causal role of *BCR-ABL* in CML (4). However, most in vitro studies have relied on the use of growth factor-dependent hematopoietic cell lines, whereas most in vivo studies have used *BCR-ABL* genes linked to strong promoters. Despite the ample literature on the mechanisms of *BCR-ABL*-induced transformation, the paucity of data in human hematopoietic progenitors from chronic and blastic phase CML and the limitations of the existing murine models leave many open questions regarding the relevant effects of *BCR-ABL* in blastic transformation of CML cells.

Ectopic expression of *BCR-ABL* in growth factor-dependent cell lines leads to the activation of numerous signal transduction pathways responsible for growth factor independence, reduced susceptibility to apoptosis, and differentiation arrest of these cells (reviewed in Ref. 1). The pleiotropic effect of *BCR-ABL* in chronic phase CML depends on post-translational modifications (i.e., phosphorylation) of signaling molecules [e.g., RAS/mitogen-activated protein kinase (MAPK), phosphatidylinositol-3 kinase (PI-3K/Akt), and signal transducers and activators of transcription (STATs) that control cell growth and survival of hematopoietic cells by modulating the expression and/or activity of downstream effectors (19). In blast crisis, increased expression of *BCR-ABL* accounts not only for activation of pathways transducing mitogenic and anti-apoptotic signals, but also for the block of differentiation, inactivation of factors with tumor suppressor activity, decreased genomic stability, and increased self-renewal of the Ph[1] blasts (15,20–23). Thus, dependence on *BCR-ABL* expression is not only a characteristic of chronic phase, but also of blast crisis CML. However, *BCR-ABL*-independent mechanisms also seem to contribute to disease progression and imatinib resistance in some CML cases (24). For example, Src kinases (e.g., Lyn) are activated in blast crisis CML (25) and appear to be responsible for a *BCR-ABL* kinase-independent mechanism of imatinib resistance (24,26) that, in part, involves Lyn-dependent induction of Bcl-2 (27). Indeed, some blast crisis patient-derived cell lines with no amplification or overexpression of wild type *BCR-ABL* are sensitive to the effect of drugs inhibiting the activity of src kinases (24,26). Nevertheless, activation of Src kinase does not seem to be required for induction of CML in mice (28).

In contrast, PI-3K and the STAT5 are important pathways required for *BCR-ABL* transformation and activated in both chronic and blastic phase CML (29,30). *BCR-ABL* interacts indirectly with the p85 regulatory subunit of PI-3K via various docking proteins, including GRB-2/Gab2 and c-cbl (31). The PI-3K activation via the GRB-2/Gab2 interaction appears pathologically relevant, as Gab2-deficient marrow cells are resistant to *BCR-ABL* transformation (31). Activation of the PI-3K pathway triggers an Akt-dependent cascade that has a critical role in *BCR-ABL* transformation and survival of $BCR-ABL^+$ myeloid progenitors (32) by regulation of the subcellular localization and/or activity of several targets, such as BAD, MDM2, IκB-kinase-α, and members of the Forkhead family of transcription factors (33). Consistent with the effects of Akt on many targets, inhibition of the PI-3K/Akt pathway suppresses in vitro colony formation and in vivo leukemogenesis of *BCR-ABL*-expressing cells (29,32), and marrow cells defective in PI-3K/Akt activation are resistant to *BCR-ABL* transformation (31). Likewise, several observations suggest the importance of STAT5 in CML. In fact (*i*) *BCR-ABL* mutants defective in STAT5 activation were less efficient than the wild-type form in the transformation of 32Dcl3 myeloid precursor cells (34); (*ii*) a constitutively active STAT5 mutant rescued the leukemogenic potential of STAT5 activation-deficient *BCR-ABL* mutants (34); and (*iii*) ectopic expression of a dominant-negative STAT5 mutant suppressed *BCR-ABL*-dependent transformation of primary mouse marrow cells (34). Furthermore, expression of p210 *BCR-ABL* in primary murine STAT5A-deficient bone marrow cells, which do not have deficiencies in colony formation, induced a B-ALL or a CML/B-ALL rather than a pure CML chronic phase-like disease in recipient mice (35), suggesting that STA5A is important for *BCR-ABL*-dependent transformation and development of a CML but not a B-ALL-like disease in mice.

Another important signal cascade in CML is the RAS pathway that becomes constitutively activated by alternative mechanisms involving the interaction of *BCR-ABL* with the GRB-2/Gab2 complex (18). The importance of RAS-dependent signaling for the phenotype of *BCR-ABL*-expressing cells is supported by the observation that downregulation of this pathway by expression of dominant-negative molecules or chemical inhibitors suppresses proliferation and sensitizes cells to apoptotic stimuli (36,37). However, it is unclear whether RAS activation leads to phosphorylation and activation of downstream signaling proteins belonging to the MAPK pathway in chronic phase CML progenitors. In contrast, compelling evidence indicates that, in hematopoietic cell lines, *BCR-ABL* expression enhances gene transcription and leads to uncontrolled generation of mitogenic and survival signals (1,18,19) in part by constitutive activation of the MEK1/2-MAPK (ERK1/2) pathway through RAS and recruitment of the serine threonine kinase Raf (1,18,19). Because neither growth factor independence nor proliferation advantage is a feature of chronic phase CML progenitors, the importance of MAPK (ERK) activation by *BCR-ABL* for the development and maintenance of CML is still unclear. Interestingly, MAPK (ERK) activity increases upon imatinib treatment as a consequence of enhanced response of CML CD34$^+$ progenitors to cytokine stimulation (38). Moreover, in the absence of exogenous cytokines, levels of activated MAPK were similar in normal and CML cells, and imatinib either reduced or did not alter MAPK activity in both normal and CML CD34$^+$ cells (38). Thus, constitutive MAPK activation does not seem to occur in primary CML progenitors, which are still capable to transiently activate MAPK in response to mitogenic and survival stimuli by extracellular growth factors (38). In fact, activation of MAPK (ERK1/2) is readily detectable in CD34$^+$ CML blast crisis, but not in CD34$^+$ CML chronic phase or CD34$^+$ normal myeloid progenitors (39). Interestingly, ERK1/2 activation appears to depend on levels of *BCR-ABL* activity, as graded *BCR-ABL* expression correlates with a progressive increase in MAPK (ERK) activity (39). Together with the ability of clinically relevant MEK1/2 inhibitors (e.g., CI-1040) to suppress proliferation and induce apoptosis of *BCR-ABL*$^+$ hematopoietic cells (40), these findings suggest that constitutive MAPK activation is essential for transduction of mitogenic, survival and, perhaps, antidifferentiation signals in blast crisis CML progenitors. In this scenario, different levels of MAPK activity may affect distinct pathways in chronic and blastic phase CML progenitors.

Although most of the data on the antiapoptotic and mitogenic pathways regulated by *BCR-ABL* have been obtained in established cell lines and may not entirely apply to primary CML cells, it is likely that most, if not all, of these pathways are less efficiently activated in primary CML cells (perhaps as a consequence of reduced *BCR-ABL* levels), but are still involved in their enhanced survival.

BCR-ABL-DEPENDENT MECHANISMS OF CHRONIC MYELOID LEUKEMIA PROGRESSION

Cytogenetic and molecular changes occur in the vast majority of CML patients during transition to blast crisis; however, the mechanism(s) whereby each specific secondary genetic alteration contributes to disease progression is still largely unclear (Fig. 2) (reviewed in Ref. 1) .

Conversely, growing evidence supports the importance of *BCR-ABL* in determining the phenotype of CML-BC cells (1), as increased *BCR-ABL* expression is a feature of CML-BC progenitors (1,15), and unrestrained *BCR-ABL* activity in CML-BC alters the expression of genes important for proliferation, survival, and maturation of myeloid progenitors (1). The cytogenetic and molecular changes observed in blast crisis CML might also be caused by the reported ability of the *BCR-ABL* oncoprotein to increase genomic instability (21,41).

Impaired Differentiation in Blast Crisis Chronic Myeloid Leukemia: Loss of C/EBPα and C/EBPβ Expression

The inability of blast crisis CML-BC myeloid progenitors to undergo terminal differentiation primarily depends on marked downregulation of C/EBPα (20), a basic region leucine zipper transcription regulator essential for granulocytic differentiation (refer Ref. 20 and the references therein). The importance of loss of C/EBPα activity as a central mechanism leading to differentiation arrest of CML myeloid blasts is supported by three lines of evidence: (*i*) ectopic C/EBPα expression induces maturation of differentiation-arrested *BCR-ABL*-expressing myeloid

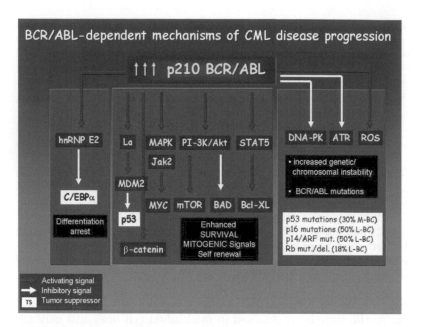

FIGURE 2 *BCR-ABL*-dependent mechanisms of chronic myeloid leukemia (CML)-disease progression. Effects of increased *BCR-ABL* expression and activity on downstream targets modulating differentiation, proliferation, survival, and genomic stability of CML progenitors. *Abbreviations*: ATR, ataxia teleoegectasia related; ROS, reactive oxygen species.

precursors (20); (*ii*) a blast crisis-like process emerges in mice transplanted with *BCR-ABL*-transduced *Cebpa*-null, but not heterozygous or wild type fetal liver cells (42); and (*iii*) genetic or functional inactivation of C/EBPα is a common event in differentiation-arrested acute myeloid leukemia blasts (reviewed in Ref. 43). In *BCR-ABL*-expressing myeloid progenitor cells, loss of C/EBPα depends on the *BCR-ABL*-induced activity of the RNA binding protein hnRNP E2 that, upon interaction with the 5′ untranslated region of *CEBPA* mRNA, inhibits *CEBPA* translation (20). In fact, the C/EBPα protein but not mRNA expression is downmodulated in primary bone marrow cells from CML-BC patients and inversely correlates with *BCR-ABL* levels (20), suggesting that the effects are dose-dependent. Accordingly, the hnRNP E2 expression is inversely correlated with that of C/EBPα (23), as hnRNP E2 levels were abundant in CML-blast crisis but undetectable in CML-chronic phase mononuclear marrow cells.

Like C/EBPα, C/EBPβ is a transcription regulator that controls myeloid maturation and a functional equivalent of C/EBPα based on its ability to restore granulocytic differentiation in C/EBPα null mice (44). In *BCR-ABL*-expressing cells, imatinib treatment shifts c/ebpβ mRNA onto polysomes. The effect of imatinib is mediated by the activity of the RNA binding protein CUGBP1 that binds a CUG-repeat region located between the first and the third AUG of c/ebpβ mRNA (45). Like C/EBPα, expression of C/EBPβ is repressed in primary CML blast crisis progenitors (45), suggesting that loss of C/EBPα and C/EBPβ activity contributes to differentiation arrest and aggressive behavior of CML blast crisis cells. Accordingly, levels of CUGBP1 were higher in normal and CML chronic phase CD34$^+$ cells than in CML blast crisis CD34$^+$ progenitors (45). Ectopic expression or inducible activation of C/EBPβ inhibits proliferation and promotes granulocytic maturation of differentiation-arrested murine *BCR-ABL*$^+$ cells through a mechanism that depends on C/EBPβ transcriptional activity (45). Thus, the antileukemic effects of C/EBPβ suggest that enhanced C/EBPβ expression might contribute to the cytotoxic effects of imatinib. Because transition to blast crisis is associated with accumulation of genetic abnormalities (i.e., loss of p53 function) and changes in gene expression (i.e., down-modulation of C/EBPα and C/EBPβ) (20,45), c-Hyc, the cellular homologue of the myelocytomatosis virus a complete loss of C/EBPs activity might be necessary to disrupt the differentiation potential of CML blast crisis progenitors.

Positive Regulation of MYC Expression

The oncogene *MYC* was one of the first identified *BCR-ABL* targets required for *BCR-ABL* leukemogenesis (46,47). Although in some blast crisis CML patients the *MYC* gene is amplified (2), several *BCR-ABL*-dependent mechanisms seem to enhance MYC expression at the transcriptional, translational, or post-translational level (39,46,48–51). One of the *BCR-ABL* pathways regulating MYC expression involves the KH-domain RNA binding protein HNRPK (hnRNP K) (39), a known transcriptional and translational regulator of gene expression (refer ref. 39 and the references therein).

In *BCR-ABL*-expressing myeloid and lymphoid progenitor cells and in CML-BC^{CD34+} but not CML-CP^{CD34+} patient cells, *BCR-ABL* kinase activity induces HNRPK expression by enhancing Hnrpk gene transcription and mRNA stability through a mechanism that depends on the *BCR-ABL*-regulated activity of MAPK$^{ERK1/2}$ (39). In fact, *BCR-ABL* graded expression activates MAPK$^{ERK1/2}$ and increases HNRPK levels in a dose-dependent manner. Knockdown of the RNA binding protein HNRPK inhibits growth factor-independent proliferation, colony formation, and tumorigenesis of *BCR-ABL*-expressing myeloid progenitors (39). Interestingly, HNRPK downregulation reduces levels of Myc (39), which is transcriptionally and translationally induced by HNRPK (52,53). In *BCR-ABL*-transformed cells, HNRPK translation-regulatory activity, which depends on phosphorylation of HNRPK on serines 284 and 353 by the *BCR-ABL*-activated MAPK$^{ERK1/2}$, is necessary for cytokine-independent proliferation, colony formation, and in vivo *BCR-ABL* leukemogenic potential of the 32D-*BCR-ABL* cell line and/or of primary CD34$^+$ CML-BC (39). The requirement of HNRPK for *BCR-ABL* leukemogenesis depends in part on its ability to bind the IRES element of MYC mRNA and enhance MYC mRNA translation (39). In fact, restoration of MYC expression is sufficient to rescue factor-independent colony formation and leukemogenic potential of 32D-*BCR-ABL* and primary CD34$^+$ CML-BC cells from the inhibitory effects of dominant-negative S284/353A HNRPK (39). Consistent with the existence of a *BCR-ABL*-MAPK-HNRPK network positively regulating MYC mRNA translation in the advanced phase of CML, MYC protein but not mRNA expression is higher in the CD34$^+$ fraction of CML-BC and -AP marrow cells than in the CD34$^+$ fraction of normal and CML-CP patient marrow cells (39). Thus, one of the molecular mechanisms whereby *BCR-ABL* enhances MYC expression involves the MAPK-dependent regulation of HNRPK translation regulatory activity. However, increased MYC mRNA levels can be still found in CML-BC patients with amplification of the MYC gene (54,55), and transcriptional, translational, and post-translational mechanisms like those involving the activity of Jak2 kinase (48) may all participate in the regulation of MYC expression in primary CML blast crisis cells.

Enhancement of MDM2 Expression as a Mechanism that Functionally Inactivates p53 in Blast Crisis Chronic Myeloid Leukemia

In *BCR-ABL*-expressing cells, the La antigen was identified as the protein that upon binding to the intercistronic region of mdm2 mRNA enhances its translation (refer ref. 22 and the references therein). Expression of the RNA binding protein La is markedly increased by *BCR-ABL* and correlated with that of MDM2 (22). La is more abundant in CML blast crisis than chronic phase primary samples and its levels appear to correlate with *BCR-ABL* levels and tyrosine kinase activity (22). Interestingly, La is a bona fide positive regulator of mdm2 translation because (*i*) it recognizes a specific conserved sequence in mdm2 mRNA that is required for efficient MDM2 expression in vitro and in vivo; (*ii*) a dominant-negative La mutant inhibited mdm2 mRNA translation in vitro and suppressed MDM2 levels in *BCR-ABL*-expressing cells; (*iii*) downregulation of La expression by siRNAs led to a marked decrease in MDM2 levels; and (*iv*) overexpression of wild-type La led to an increase in MDM2 expression (22). That La-mediated effect on MDM2 expression is functionally relevant for *BCR-ABL* leukemogenesis is indicated by the changes in susceptibility of *BCR-ABL*-expressing cells to adriamycin-induced apoptosis, as wild-type La-overexpressing cells were more resistant than parental cells, whereas cells expressing dominant negative La were more sensitive (22). Although MDM2 levels were markedly downmodulated in *BCR-ABL* cells expressing the dominant-negative La, these cells neither exhibited spontaneous apoptosis nor altered cell cycle activity, consistent with the primary role of MDM2 as a negative regulator of p53. Inactivating mutations of the p53 gene are rarely found in chronic phase, but are relatively common in blast crisis (56), suggesting that loss of function of p53 plays an important role in disease progression. Indeed, loss of wild-type p53 potentiates the leukemia-inducing effects of *BCR-ABL*, as indicated by the rapidly fatal disease process induced in recipient mice by transplantation of *BCR-ABL*-expressing p53-deficient marrow cells (57,58). Since genetic inactivation of p53 is detected in approximately 25% of CML-BC patients (56), the La-dependent induction of MDM2 expression may represent a mechanism whereby *BCR-ABL* functionally inactivates p53 in CML blast crisis patients with a wild-type p53 gene. Indeed, p53 expression is inhibited by ectopic *BCR-ABL* expression in myeloid progenitor 32Dcl3 cells through a mechanism that does not involve expression of p19ARF, but depends on increased expression of MDM2 and can be reverted by inhibition of the proteasome activity (22). Thus, the La-dependent translational stimulation of MDM2 expression not only might be relevant for survival of CML blast crisis progenitors, but may also contribute to disease progression through functional inactivation of the p53 tumor suppressor.

Loss of PP2A Tumor Suppressor Activity in Blast Crisis Chronic Myeloid Leukemia: A *BCR-ABL* Auto-Protective and Gain-of-Function Mechanism

In CML blast crisis, PP2A inactivation results from increased expression of SET, a physiological inhibitor of PP2A, which is induced by *BCR-ABL* in a dose- and kinase-dependent manner and, like *BCR-ABL*, progressively increases during transition to blast crisis (23). Interestingly, increased SET expression like that of Bcl-X$_L$ seems to depend on the increased mRNA export activity of hnRNP A1, an RNA binding protein overexpressed in CML blast crisis and required for cytokine-independent proliferation, survival, and leukemogenesis of acute phase CML blasts and *BCR-ABL*-expressing myeloid progenitor cell lines (59).

The tumor suppressing activity of the PP2A serine/threonine phosphatase depends on its ability to dephosphorylate several factors implicated in the regulation of cell cycle, proliferation, survival, and differentiation. Remarkably, several targets are shared by *BCR-ABL* and PP2A. Among these, expression and/or activity of certain PP2A substrates are either essential for *BCR-ABL* leukemogenesis or have been found altered in CML-BC (refer ref. 23 and the references therein). In *BCR-ABL$^+$* myeloid progenitor 32Dcl3 cells, SET downregulation and forced expression of PP2Ac suppress MAPK, STAT5, and Akt phosphorylation, decreases Myc expression, and increases levels of pro-apoptotic BAD and of hypophosphorylated Rb. Since ectopic SET expression antagonizes the effects of exogenous PP2A (23), SET-dependent suppression of PP2A activity may represent one of the mechanisms used by *BCR-ABL* to prevent inactivation of mitogenic and survival signals in CML blast crisis progenitors.

In imatinib-sensitive and -resistant (T315I included) *BCR-ABL* cell lines and in CML-BC^{CD34+} patient cells, restoration of PP2A phosphatase activity, either by chemical PP2A activators or by interfering with the SET/PP2A interplay, promotes *BCR-ABL* tyrosine dephosphorylation (inactivation) which, in turn, trigger its proteasome-dependent degradation (23). Mechanistically, *BCR-ABL* proteolysis appears to depend on the PP2A-induced activation of the tumor suppressor SHP-1 tyrosine phosphatase and on the coexistence of *BCR-ABL*, PP2A, and SHP-1 in the same multiprotein complex (23). In fact, increased cytokine-independent clonogenic potential and inability of PP2A to promote *BCR-ABL* degradation was observed in *BCR-ABL*-transduced SHP-1-decifient lineage-negative marrow myeloid progenitors cells (23). The involvement of SHP-1 in the PP2A-induced negative regulation of *BCR-ABL* kinase activity and expression is also supported by the fact that SHP-1 associates with *BCR-ABL*, and its tyrosine phosphatase activity counteracts *BCR-ABL* leukemogenic potential (60). Accordingly, expression of SHP-1 is diminished in most leukemias and lymphomas, its downregulation leads to abnormal cell growth, and its activity is suppressed by different oncogenic tyrosine kinases (e.g., FLT3/ITD and JAK) (61–63). Thus, functional inactivation of PP2A by increased *BCR-ABL* kinase activity seems to be required for the transduction of aberrant mitogenic, survival and antidifferentiation signals, and for the post-translational enhancement of *BCR-ABL* expression and oncogenic activity in CML-BC^{CD34+} marrow myeloid progenitors. Restoring normal PP2A activity induces marked apoptosis, reduces proliferation, impairs colony formation, inhibits tumorigenesis, and promotes differentiation of wild type, Y253H and T315I *BCR-ABL$^+$* cell lines and primary blast crisis CD34$^+$ CML cells (23). Importantly, in vivo administration of the PP2A activators forskolin or 1,9-dideoxy forskolin also markedly suppresses the development of wild type and T315I *BCR-ABL*-induced CML blast crisis-like disease without exerting significant adverse effects on normal hematopoiesis (23). Because of the central role of PP2A in the regulation of cell growth, survival and differentiation, its loss-of-function most likely contributes to blastic transformation of CML.

Effect of *BCR-ABL* on DNA Repair and Genomic Stability

The transition of CML from chronic phase to blast crisis is characterized by the accumulation of molecular and chromosomal abnormalities (64), but the molecular mechanisms underlying this genetic instability are poorly understood (65). In the past two to three years, few studies have directly addressed the relationship between *BCR-ABL* expression and levels/activity of proteins involved in DNA repair, particularly the repair of DNA double-strand breaks (21).

In the first study investigating such a relationship, Deutsch et al. (66) looked at the effects of *BCR-ABL* on the catalytic subunit, DNA-PK$_{CS}$, of the DNA-PK complex formed with the heterodimeric Ku protein. Repair of DSBs by the DNA-PK-dependent pathway [nonhomologous end-joining (NHEJ) recombination] is the preferred pathway utilized by human cells (67), and in mice, NHEJ deficiency accelerates lymphoma formation and promotes the development of soft tissue sarcomas that possess clonal amplifications, deletions, and translocations (68,69). In *BCR-ABL*-expressing cells (including primary CML cells), levels of DNA-PK$_{CS}$ were markedly downregulated (66) and were reversed by proteasome inhibitors, suggesting the activation of a *BCR-ABL*-dependent pathway leading to enhanced proteasome-dependent protein degradation (66). Downregulation of DNA-PK$_{CS}$ levels was associated with a higher frequency of chromosomal abnormalities after exposure of *BCR-ABL*-expressing cells to ionizing radiation (IR) and increased radiosensitivity (66). Such an increase was, however, modest probably due to enhanced survival of *BCR-ABL*-expressing cells caused by the activation of multiple antiapoptotic pathways. The same group also reported an association of *BCR-ABL* expression in primary CML samples and in established cell lines with downregulation of BRCA-1 (70), a protein involved in the surveillance of genome integrity (71,72). Downregulation of BRCA-1 was more evident in cell lines in which levels of *BCR-ABL* were more abundant and correlated with increased chromosome aberrations after DNA damage. However, these findings have not been yet confirmed in a large cohort of primary samples obtained from CML patients, and a causal link between decreased repair of DSBs and disease progression has not been demonstrated. Another group identified *BCR-ABL*-dependent pathways leading to enhanced expression/ activity of RAD51 (73), a protein that participates in homologous recombination repair (HRR) (74). Expression of *BCR-ABL* increased the efficiency of HRR in a RAD51-dependent manner as well as resistance to apoptosis induced by drugs like mitomycin C and cisplatin, which promote DSBs (73). In light of enhanced high-fidelity HRR promoted by RAD51 (74), it seems counterintuitive that the increased expression/ activity of RAD51 (and other paralogues) in *BCR-ABL*-expressing cells might be associated with genomic instability. Together, the apparently opposite effects of *BCR-ABL* on RAD51, DNA-PK$_{CS}$, and BRCA-1 may not be mutually exclusive and may all be involved in promoting genomic instability associated with defective repair of DSBs. Deregulation of the DNA repair mechanisms and the acquisition of mutations in genes critically important for the regulation of proliferation are expected to activate control checkpoints (i.e., p53 expression), which may lead to the elimination of cells with damaged DNA. However, the ability of *BCR-ABL* to regulate multiple antiapoptotic pathways, perhaps in a dose-dependent manner and in specific subsets of progenitor cells, is likely to allow survival of cell populations carrying mutations that promote their proliferation and maintenance. In this regard, appears to the unrestrained *BCR-ABL* kinase activity induce an increase in reactive oxygen species (ROS), which can cause chronic oxidative

DNA damage resulting in the accumulation of DSBs (75). These lesions are repaired by *BCR-ABL*-stimulated HRR and NHEJ mechanisms; however, a high mutation rate is detected in HRR, and large deletions are found in NHEJ products in *BCR-ABL*-expressing cells, but not in the normal counterparts (75). Interestingly, the *BCR-ABL*-dependent increase in the levels of oxidative DNA damage is also responsible for the emergence of clinically relevant mutations in the kinase domain of *BCR-ABL* itself (76). Conversely, Dierov et al. (77) reported that *BCR-ABL* interacts with the ATR protein (atoxic teleoegectasia related) in the nucleus and suppresses its activity, implicating this mechanism in the increased number of DSBs after etoposide treatment, and suggesting a delay in DNA double strand break repair after genotoxic stress. Furthermore, the same group has examined the occurrence of chromosomal abnormalities in *BCR-ABL* expressing cells after recovery from DNA damage (41) and found that *BCR-ABL*-transduced BaF3 cells compared to parental cells exhibit an increase in chromosomal abnormalities, including chromatid damage, after DNA repair (41). Similar studies in primary human cells show increased frequency of translocations in CML samples versus normal hematopoietic progenitors (M. Carroll, personal communication).

From the data discussed earlier, it seems that the mechanism(s) leading to increased genomic instability is(are) still not yet well defined. However, it seems likely that *BCR-ABL* expression alters the cellular response to genotoxic stress and predisposes cells to genetic (e.g., point mutations) and gross chromosomal alterations (e.g., translocations), which, undoubtedly, contribute to the aggressiveness of CML blast crisis cells.

GENETIC/MOLECULAR ABNORMALITIES IN BLAST CRISIS CHRONIC MYELOID LEUKEMIA

Cytogenetic and molecular changes occur in a vast majority of CML patients during evolution to blast crisis (reviewed in Ref. 1). Thus, a recurring question has been whether p210$^{BCR-ABL}$ induces genomic instability directly, or increasingly frequent genetic abnormalities during disease progression are acquired secondarily. Also, neither situation excludes that genetic instability of CML blast crisis depends both on increased propensity of *BCR-ABL*-expressing cells to undergo genetic changes and the probability that one of the mutations induced by *BCR-ABL* functions as an "amplifier" of a genetically unstable phenotype.

While the persistent expression of *BCR-ABL*, per se, may lead to genomic instability, there is also a cohort of CML patients (10–15%) presenting with deletions of the derivative chromosome 9, which, ab initio, may be more prone to genomic instability (78). These patients progress to blast crisis much more rapidly than CML patients lacking the deletion and develop identical chromosomal abnormalities, consistent with the proposed explanation of a genetic mechanism (loss of a tumor suppressor/modifier gene?), which accelerates a *BCR-ABL*-driven disease process (78).

The role of *BCR-ABL* in promoting genetic instability has been investigated in preleukemic transgenic mice expressing p190$^{BCR-ABL}$. Since these mice develop B-cell type acute lymphocytic leukemia at high frequency, it is unclear whether the findings may also apply to a preleukemic phase induced by p210$^{BCR-ABL}$. Nevertheless, in this mouse model of *BCR-ABL*-induced leukemia, point mutations, insertions, and deletions were detected with increased frequency in the preleukemic phase (79) and their occurrence was, in part, blocked by imatinib treatment (79).

Microsatellite instability, a feature associated with tumor progression, does not seem to be involved in CML disease progression (80). Nevertheless, 60% to 80% of CML patients develop additional nonrandom chromosomal abnormalities involving chromosomes 8, 17, 19, and 22 with duplication of the Ph chromosome or trisomy 8 being the most frequent (81).

At the molecular level, mutation of the tumor suppressor gene p53 is detected in approximately 25% to 30% of CML-myeloid blast crisis (56), whereas approximately 50% of the patients with lymphoid blast crisis present a homozygous deletion at the INK4A/ARF gene locus located on chromosome 9 (82). The most common chromosomal changes are trisomy of chromosome 8 (34%), trisomy of chromosome 19 (13%), double Ph chromosome (38%), isochromosome i(17q) (20%); these abnormalities can be also found in various combinations. On the basis of the frequency of the combinations in all metaphases and subclones, it has been suggested that i(17q) and trisomy of chromosome 8 are early changes, whereas trisomy 19 might occur late during disease progression (81). Some combinations [trisomy 8, double Ph chromosome and i(17q)] are more frequent than others; but, neither the presumed order of appearance nor the combination itself seems to have a clear impact on the prognosis of CML-BC (81). Moreover, the frequency of some secondary changes seems to depend on the therapeutic regimen (81). For example, chromosome 8 trisomy is more frequent in CML patients treated with busulfan (44%) than in those receiving hydroxyurea (12%). The frequency of the common CML secondary changes in interferon-α (IFN-α)-treated patients and especially after bone marrow transplantation appears to be lower than in the busulfan-treated group (81), suggesting that the treatment with DNA-damaging agents (i.e., busulfan) accentuates the genetic instability caused by the unrestrained tyrosine kinase activity of *BCR-ABL*. It will be interesting to see whether evolution into CML-BC of imatinib-treated CML patients is also associated with a subset of the chromosomal abnormalities found in the "historical" group of CML patients predominantly treated with busulfan and/or hydroxyurea.

Whether and how the most common chromosomal abnormalities of CML-BC are pathogenetically linked to disease progression remains unclear and difficult to prove. Interestingly, the role of the double Ph chromosome in disease progression is also unclear. Perhaps the presence of this chromosomal abnormality leads to increased expression of *BCR-ABL*, which has also been reported in advanced disease stages (1). However, the relationship between *BCR-ABL* levels and presence of the second Ph chromosome has not been formally tested. Whether the increased expression of *BCR-ABL*, per se, is sufficient to induce blast crisis is uncertain. For example, expression of *BCR-ABL* in retrovirus-transduced marrow cells is quite abundant (83) and yet mice succumb because of a myeloproliferative disorder rather than an acute leukemia with accumulation of blast cells.

Perhaps, what matters is increased and sustained expression of *BCR-ABL* in a primitive pool of hematopoietic progenitor cells. As extensively discussed earlier, expression of C/EBPα, which is required for myeloid differentiation (84), is down-regulated by *BCR-ABL* in a dose-dependent manner (20) and its expression restored G-CSF-induced differentiation of *BCR-ABL*-expressing cells, suggesting that C/EBPα is a critical target in CML disease progression (20). Similarly, increased expression of *BCR-ABL* in blast crisis CML is responsible for the inactivation of PP2A phosphatase that, when reactivated, impairs *BCR-ABL* signaling and promotes inactivation and degradation of *BCR-ABL* itself (23). Few genes upregulated in CML-BC may be involved in disease progression in patients with double Ph chromosome. Two of such genes are mdm2 and MYC, which are activated by *BCR-ABL* post-transcriptionally (22,39) and function by halting the p53-mediated DNA damage response and transducing mitogenic/survival signals, respectively.

Two other genes upregulated by *BCR-ABL* in CML-BC are Evi-1 and HOXA9, two transcription factors which can cooperate with *BCR-ABL* in blocking myeloid differentiation and enhancing the proliferative and survival advantage of *BCR-ABL*-expressing cells (85,86). Perhaps, the cumulative effect of MYC, mdm2, Evi-1, HoxA9, and other *BCR-ABL* targets involved in proliferation, survival and differentiation coupled with loss of PP2A tumor suppressor activity and downregulation of C/EBPα leads incrementally to differentiation arrest, reduced apoptosis susceptibility, and enhanced proliferative potential of CML blast crisis cells.

That there are *BCR-ABL* dose-dependent mechanisms of altered gene regulation, clearly not limited to those described, might be important to explain the disease process of blast crisis CML without chromosomal and molecular abnormalities and the relative sensitivity to imatinib of blast crisis cells. In fact, $\sim$30% (preimatinib era) (81,87) and $\sim$50% (postimatinib era) (88) of CML-BC patients do not exhibit chromosomal abnormalities and presumably only a fraction of these patients has molecular inactivation of the p53 gene, and yet their overall survival is only marginally better of those with chromosomal abnormalities. It is tempting to speculate that the disease burden of patients without chromosomal abnormalities is a consequence of the epigenetic changes (i.e., inactivation of PP2A, downmodulation of C/EBPα, and increased MDM2 and MYC levels) induced by *BCR-ABL* overexpression. The therapeutic response of CML-BC patients to imatinib may be, in part, also explained by suppression of the dosage-dependent effects of *BCR-ABL*, which are likely to coexist with the effects of chromosomal and molecular abnormalities. Inhibition of *BCR-ABL* activity is not expected to reverse the effects of the chromosomal and molecular abnormalities of CML blast crisis cells, while the consequences of *BCR-ABL* dose-dependent effects on gene expression would be reversed, at least until the emergence of cell subpopulations with mutant *BCR-ABL*, a process which may be also favored by *BCR-ABL* overexpression (17,76).

Overexpression of *BCR-ABL* might be also involved in transcriptional repression by promoting hypermethylation of the regulatory regions of specific genes. One such gene is c-Abl itself, which is hypermethylated and expressed at low levels in CML-BC (89). The c-Abl protein has been implicated in the DNA damage response and in apoptosis (90); thus, downmodulation of c-Abl expression might further reduce susceptibility to DNA-damage-induced apoptosis of *BCR-ABL* expressing cells while enhancing their genomic instability, two features that can contribute to disease progression. The involvement of c-Abl loss in disease progression remains speculative because it has not been tested yet in any in vitro or in vivo model of *BCR-ABL*-dependent transformation of hematopoietic cells.

The most common gene mutations in CML-blast crisis involve the p53 gene (which is mutated in 25–30% of myeloid CML-blast crisis) and the INK4A/ARF exon 2 (which is homozygously deleted in approximately 50% of lymphoid CML-BC). The pathogenic role of p53 loss of function in CML disease progression has been tested using two different strategies. We showed that mice injected with p53-deficient, *BCR-ABL*-expressing marrow cells developed a more aggressive disease process than those injected with wild-type p53, *BCR-ABL*-expressing marrow cells (58). Compared to p53 wild-type cells, p53-deficient *BCR-ABL*-expressing marrow cells were morphologically undifferentiated, more resistant to apoptosis induced by growth factor deprivation, and highly clonogenic in growth factor-deprived cultures (58). Blastic transformation of marrow cells was also obtained in a transgenic model in which mice expressing p210$^{BCR-ABL}$ under the control of the Tec promoter were crossed with p53-heterozygous (p53+/−) mice (57). The *BCR-ABL*+/−, p53+/− mice died of acute leukemia, which was preceded by a myeloproliferative disorder resembling human CML. Interestingly, the residual normal p53 allele of *BCR-ABL*-expressing blast cells was frequently lost, implying the existence of a *BCR-ABL*-dependent mechanism facilitating loss of the remaining p53 allele. One interpretation of these findings is that *BCR-ABL* accelerates the tumorigenic conversion of cells prone to transformation by inactivation of one p53 allele.

Despite the absence of an ideal in vivo model testing the role of p53 loss of function in myeloid blast crisis, p53 loss can contribute to disease progression in several ways. Compared to wild-type marrows, p53−/− cells showed a three- to four-fold increase in the frequency of multipotent progenitors (Lin⁻Sca-1⁺, CD34⁺) and a greater number of hematopoietic stem cells capable of hematopoietic reconstitution in lethally irradiated mice (91). Moreover, these cells were less susceptible to apoptotic stimuli (91). Lineage commitment and differentiation of p53−/− progenitors was not affected, suggesting that loss of p53, per se, does not cause differentiation arrest (91). Thus, the differentiation arrest of CML blast crisis cells lacking a functional p53 gene may be due to the effect of *BCR-ABL* in an expanded pool of hematopoietic progenitors and/or secondary mutations induced by the cumulative effects of *BCR-ABL* and p53 loss of function in promoting genomic instability.

Another common mutation in CML-blast crisis is homozygous deletion of exon 2 at the INK4A/ARF locus. The frequency of this mutation is approximately 50% in lymphoid blast crisis, but is undetectable in myeloid blast crisis (82,92). Exon 2 deletion of the INK4A/ARF locus is expected to result in loss of expression of p16 and p14/ARF, two proteins that regulate cell cycle progression and the G1/S checkpoint by inhibiting the G1 phase cyclin D-Cdk4/Cdk6 and promoting p53 upregulation, respectively. The involvement of p16 and ARF in the maintenance of adult self-renewing hematopoietic stem cells has recently been suggested by a study in which ectopic expression of p16 or ARF in hematopoietic stem cells (c-Kit⁺, Sca-1⁺, and Flt3⁻Lin⁻) suppressed their proliferation, with ARF being more potent than p16 (93). Thus, it is likely that loss of p16 and ARF-dependent p53 activities are both necessary for lymphoid transformation in the subset of CML-blast crisis patients with homozygous deletion of the p16/ARF locus. However, the relative contribution of p16 and ARF is unknown. On the basis of the relationship between ARF and p53 expression, where ARF induces increased p53 levels by interfering with its MDM2-dependent degradation (94), homozygous deletion at the p16/ARF locus observed in lymphoid blast crisis might represent a functional equivalent of p53 mutation in myeloid blast crisis. However, ARF appears to have also p53-independent effects (95), which could contribute to the phenotype of lymphoid blast crisis cells. Loss of p16INK4A leads indirectly to abrogation/attenuation of the cell cycle regulatory effects of the p105 retinoblastoma protein (RB); however, the Rb gene itself is often inactivated in the accelerated or blast crisis phase of CML especially that associated with a megakaryoblastic or lymphoblastic phenotype (96). Rb is inactivated by mutation, deletion, or loss of expression in approximately 18% of CML blast crisis cases.

A UNIFYING MECHANISM FOR DISEASE PROGRESSION
IN CHRONIC MYELOID LEUKEMIA

As discussed earlier, CML blast crisis is characterized by a number of seemingly incoherent chromosomal and molecular abnormalities and by a cascade of effects deriving from the increased activity of p210 *BCR-ABL* oncoprotein. Yet, some generalizations can be attempted:

1. the vast majority of secondary changes involve genes encoding nucleus-localized proteins that directly or indirectly regulate gene transcription;
2. inactivating mutations/loss-of-function of tumor suppressor genes are more common than activating mutation/gain-of-function of oncogenes; and
3. p53 is genetically or functionally inactivated in a large fraction of CML-blast crisis.

Vis-a-vis the central role of the cytoplasm-localized *BCR-ABL* in disease initiation and progression, it is not surprising that most secondary changes of CML blast crisis involve genes encoding nucleus-localized proteins. The *BCR-ABL* oncoprotein activates several signal transduction pathways regulating cell proliferation and survival, and additional mutations activating these pathways would be of no obvious advantage. Indeed, mutation of K-RAS or N-RAS is a rare event in CML blast crisis, and mutation of PTEN, which is frequent in solid tumors and leads to constitutive activation of the PI-3K/Akt pathway, has not been detected in any leukemia sample, including CML (reviewed in Ref. 1). Thus, mutations of nucleus-localized gene products can be seen as complementing the effects of the cytoplasm-localized *BCR-ABL*. Among the nucleus-localized gene products mutated in CML blast crisis, some activate or repress transcription directly (NOP98/HOXA9 and AML-1/EVI-1, respectively), some lead to a nonfunctional transcription factor (i.e., p53 mutant), and some indirectly modulate the activity of transcription factors involved in DNA synthesis (i.e., homozygous deletions of the p16INK4A/ARF locus leading to inactivation of the Rb pathway and enhanced activity of E2F family genes) or in cell cycle checkpoints (i.e., homozygous deletions of the p16INK4A/ARF locus leading to MDM2-dependent inactivation/degradation of p53). Regardless of the predominant secondary change(s) of CML blast crisis, in any of the above situations, the phenotype is remarkably similar and consists of growth factor-independent proliferation and survival coexisting with a severe differentiation arrest. The most likely interpretation of these findings is that the differentiation arrest of CML blast crisis cells can be enforced by mutations/downregulation of differentiation-regulatory genes (i.e., generation of the AML-1/EVI-1 chimera or reduced C/EBPα expression), as well as by activation of proliferation-stimulatory pathways (i.e., homozygous deletion of the p16INK4A/ARF locus with secondary effects on the Rb and p53 pathway, and PP2A inactivation with consequent enhancement of mitogenic and survival signals). In addition, loss of PP2A tumor suppressor activity (23) most likely contributes to increased self-renewal and expansion of the blast crisis CML leukemia-initiating cell by preventing β-catenin degradation (97) and, therefore, enhancing WNT/β-catenin signaling (Fig. 3) (15).

In many cell types, differentiation is preceded by reduced proliferation, and an abnormally high proliferative rate in a specific stem/progenitor cell subset might lead to expansion of a cell population unfit to differentiate. Most secondary genetic abnormalities in CML blast crisis directly inactivate genes that function as

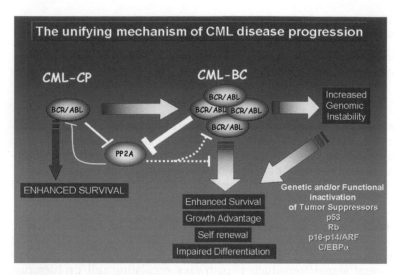

FIGURE 3   A unifying mechanism of chronic myeloid leukemia (CML) disease progression. A model of CML disease progression resulting from the combined effects of *BCR-ABL* overexpression and *BCR-ABL*-dependent genomic instability. In this unifying model of disease progression that sees *BCR-ABL* as the key-player, the tumor suppressor PP2A will have the role of a "gatekeeper," as its activation controls and restrains *BCR-ABL* expression/activity, whereas its inhibition allows *BCR-ABL* expression to increase and induce a cascade of events that promote disease progression by enhancing survival, proliferation and self renewal, impairing differentiation and increasing genomic instability of a CD34$^+$ CML cell clone. *Abbreviations*: CML, chronic myeloid leukemia; CML-CP, chronic myeloid leukemia-chronic phase; CML-BC, chronic myeloid leukemia-blast crisis.

tumor suppressors (i.e., p53 gene mutations) or lead to functional inactivation of tumor suppressor genes (i.e., homozygous deletion of ARF leading to p53 loss of function). In this regard, CML disease progression is similar to the transition from a premalignant to a frank neoplastic state in solid tumors. In contrast to CML and other hematological malignancies, in solid tumors the initiating event is often represented by inactivation of a tumor suppressor gene.

Genetic or functional inactivation of p53 seems the most common abnormality in CML blast crisis, as the p53 gene is mutated in 25% to 30% of myeloid CML blast crisis. Homozygous deletion of the p16INK4A/ARF locus, which indirectly affects p53 function, is detected in approximately 50% of CML lymphoid blast crisis, and expression of MDM2, the principal negative regulator of p53, is often more abundant in CML blast crisis mononuclear cells, compared to the corresponding chronic phase cells (22). Other mechanisms potentially leading to functional inactivation of p53 (i.e., cytoplasmic sequestration) have not been examined, making difficult a quantitation of the actual involvement of p53 in CML disease progression. In this regard, no studies have addressed directly the issue of functional inactivation of p53 in CML disease progression, and an assessment of the frequency of this mechanism seems necessary.

CONCLUSIONS

A legitimate model of disease progression in CML predicts that *BCR-ABL* activity promotes the accumulation of genetic and epigenetic alterations directly or indirectly responsible for the reduced apoptosis susceptibility and the enhanced proliferative potential and differentiation arrest of CML blast crisis cells. Indeed, there is evidence for a mechanism of CML disease progression where alterations in DNA repair processes coupled with enhanced survival of *BCR-ABL*-expressing cells may allow the propagation of secondary genetic changes that favor the emergence and persistence of increasingly malignant cells. Among the secondary changes, those directly or indirectly affecting the p53 tumor suppressor gene seem to have a central role for frequency and biological consequences.

At the molecular level, CML blast crisis remains a heterogeneous disease and yet only few pathways are commonly affected. Of the many issues that need to be investigated for a better understanding of the pathogenic mechanisms in CML disease progression, some should attract considerable attention.

First, is *BCR-ABL* overexpression a common feature of blast crisis CML and is determined stochastically or by genetic/epigenetic mechanisms? Recent evidence suggests that expression of *BCR-ABL* is more abundant in early than in late CML chronic phase progenitors and that CML blast crisis undifferentiated and committed myeloid progenitors express higher *BCR-ABL* levels of the corresponding chronic phase progenitors (1,15,17,23). If this is confirmed by additional studies, an obvious question will be whether *BCR-ABL* overexpression is causally linked or secondary to the expansion of homogeneous populations of blast cells. A molecular characterization of apparently identical subpopulations of CML-chronic phase and blast crisis progenitors and their comparison with normal progenitors may prove important in addressing these possibilities. Overexpression of *BCR-ABL* during disease progression may be the result of stochastic forces and/or facilitated by genetic/epigenetic mechanisms. We favor the second hypothesis, as restoration of PP2A activity in myeloid CML blast crisis cells leads to SHP-1-mediated dephosphorylation and proteasome-dependent degradation of *BCR-ABL*, suggesting that functional inactivation of PP2A tumor suppressor by *BCR-ABL* represents an auto-regulatory mechanism allowing increased and sustained *BCR-ABL* activity and expression in early CML blast crisis progenitors (23). However, a more detailed analysis of the mechanisms responsible for increased *BCR-ABL* expression in CML blast crisis patients with and without chromosomal/molecular abnormalities could be informative in supporting or disproving either possibility.

Second, are there specific molecular determinants of lymphoid CML blast crisis and do they interact with *BCR-ABL* in selectively promoting the expansion of B-cell type blasts? The high frequency of homozygous deletions at the INK4A/ARF locus suggests that inactivation of the INK4A or ARF gene or both serves as the important molecular determinant of lymphoid blast crisis. Since specific knockout models (INK4A−/−, ARF−/−, and INK4A/ARF−/−) are available, it will be important to test whether INK4A, ARF, or the combination of both mutants cooperates with *BCR-ABL* to induce the selective expansion of a pool of progenitors committed to B-cell development. Perhaps, loss of the INK4A or ARF gene or both favors cell cycle entry of B-cell type rather than myeloid progenitors. Loss of p16 and ARF function is required for immortalization of human cells, whereas loss of ARF is sufficient for immortalization and RAS-dependent transformation of mouse cells (98); thus, the role of ARF and p16 should also be independently tested in in vitro models of *BCR-ABL* transformation of multipotent and unipotent human progenitor cells.

Third, will disease progression and development of secondary genetic abnormalities be affected by imatinib monotherapy? If disease progression depends on the constitutive activity of the *BCR-ABL* tyrosine kinase, suppressing its activity will postpone, if not prevent, the development of CML blast crisis. Although there is no proof for it, the secondary changes of CML blast crisis may reflect, in part, the effects of treatment with DNA damaging agents on the genetically unstable background of *BCR-ABL*-expressing cells. If so, imatinib-resistant CML blast crisis might be characterized by a distinct pattern of secondary changes primarily caused by the constitutive activity of *BCR-ABL*. It is also possible that the molecular mechanisms of disease progression will be totally different in those patients resistant to imatinib as well as to AMN107 and dasatinib (11); however, it is unclear whether the T315I is a gain-of-function mutation that confers increased kinase activity to *BCR-ABL* (99). The ultimate goal of *BCR-ABL* kinase inhibitor-based CML therapy is disease eradication and prevention of transition to blast crisis. Since it is unlikely that this will be achieved in each patient, as it appears that both imatinib and dasatinib are not effective in killing the so-called quiescent CML stem cell (8), understanding disease progression in the imatinib-resistant group will be essential for the development of "rational" therapeutic strategies [e.g., PP2A activating compounds (23) or drugs able to restore C/EBPα expression and its tumor suppressor and pro-differentiation activities (100)] to be used in conjunction with *BCR-ABL* tyrosine kinase inhibitors.

SUMMARY

CML evolves from a chronic phase characterized by Ph^1 as the sole genetic alteration to blast crisis, which is often associated with increased expression of the *BCR-ABL* oncoprotein, and with the presence of additional chromosomal and molecular abnormalities. Although the pathogenic effects of most CML blast crisis secondary changes are still poorly understood, the phenotype of CML blast crisis cells (enhanced proliferation and survival, differentiation arrest) appears to depend on co-operation of *BCR-ABL* with gene(s) that become dysregulated during disease progression.

Most genetic abnormalities of CML blast crisis have a direct or indirect effect on p53 and/or Rb gene activity, which are primarily required for cell proliferation and survival, but not differentiation. Thus, the differentiation arrest of CML blast crisis cells is a secondary consequence of these abnormalities or is caused by deregulation of differentiation-regulatory genes (i.e., C/EBPα). Furthermore, loss of PP2A tumor suppressor activity in blast crisis CML allows *BCR-ABL* to transduce aberrant mitogenic, survival and antidifferentiation signals, and enhance post-translationally its expression and oncogenic activity.

Validation of the critical role of certain secondary changes (i.e., loss of p53, PP2A, or C/EBPα function) in murine models of CML blast crisis and in in vitro assays of *BCR-ABL* transformation of human hematopoietic progenitors might lead to the development of novel therapies based on targeting *BCR-ABL* and inhibiting or restoring the gene activity gained or lost during disease progression (i.e., p53, PP2A, or C/EBPα).

ACKNOWLEDGMENTS

This work is supported in part by National Cancer Institute grants to D. Perrotti (CA095512) and B. Calabretta (CA78890) and by Department of the Army

CMLRP grants to D. Perrotti (DAMD17-03-1-0184) and to B. Calabretta (W81XWH04-1-0807).

We apologize in advance to those investigators whose work or contributions were not cited due to space limitations.

REFERENCES

1. Calabretta Perrotti D. The biology of CML blast crisis. Blood 2004; 103:4010–4022.
2. Melo, JV. The molecular biology of chronic myeloid leukaemia. Leukemia 1996; 10:751–756.
3. Daley GQ, Baltimore D. Transformation of an interleukin 3-dependent hematopoietic cell line by the chronic myelogenous leukemia-specific P210BCR-ABL protein. Proc Natl Acad Sci USA 1998; 85:9312–9316.
4. Daley GQ, Van Etten RA, Baltimore D. Induction of chronic myelogenous leukemia in mice by the P210bcr/abl gene of the Philadelphia chromosome. Science 1990; 247:824–830.
5. Weisdorf DJ, et al. Allogeneic bone marrow transplantation for chronic myelogenous leukemia: comparative analysis of unrelated versus matched sibling donor transplantation. Blood 2002; 99:1971–1977.
6. Deininger M, Buchdunger E, Druker BJ. The development of imatinib as a therapeutic agent for chronic myeloid leukemia. Blood 2005; 105:2640–2653.
7. Hughes TP, et al. Frequency of major molecular responses to imatinib or interferon alfa plus cytarabine in newly diagnosed chronic myeloid leukemia. N Engl J Med 2003; 349:1423–1432.
8. Copland M, et al. Dasatinib (BMS-354825) targets an earlier progenitor population than imatinib in primary CML, but does not eliminate the quiescent fraction. Blood 2006.
9. Shah NP, Sawyers CL. Mechanisms of resistance to STI571 in Philadelphia chromosome-associated leukemias. Oncogene 2003; 22:7389–7395.
10. Walz C, Sattler M. Novel targeted therapies to overcome imatinib mesylate resistance in chronic myeloid leukemia (CML). Crit Rev Oncol Hematol 2006; 57:145–164.
11. O'Hare T, et al. In vitro activity of Bcr-Abl inhibitors AMN107 and BMS-354825 against clinically relevant imatinib-resistant Abl kinase domain mutants. Cancer Res 2005; 65:4500–4505.
12. Deininger MWN, et al. Comparison of imatinib, AMN107 and dasatinib in an accelerated cell-based mutagenesis screen. Blood 2005; 106:691.
13. Gaiger A, et al. Increase of bcr-abl chimeric mRNA expression in tumor cells of patients with chronic myeloid leukemia precedes disease progression. Blood 1995; 86:2371–2378.
14. Schultheis B, Szydlo R, Mahon FX, Apperley JF, Melo JV. Analysis of total phosphotyrosine levels in CD34+ cells from CML patients to predict the response to imatinib mesylate treatment. Blood 2005; 105:4893–4894.
15. Jamieson CH, et al. Granulocyte-macrophage progenitors as candidate leukemic stem cells in blast-crisis CML. N Engl J Med 2004; 351:657–667.
16. Soverini S, et al. ABL mutations in late chronic phase chronic myeloid leukemia patients with up-front cytogenetic resistance to imatinib are associated with a greater likelihood of progression to blast crisis and shorter survival: a study by the GIMEMA Working Party on chronic myeloid leukemia. J Clin Oncol 2005; 23:4100–4109.
17. Barnes DJ, et al. Bcr-Abl expression levels determine the rate of development of resistance to imatinib mesylate in chronic myeloid leukemia. Cancer Res 2005; 65:8912–8919.
18. Arlinghaus R, Sun T. Signal transduction pathways in Bcr-Abl transformed cells. Cancer Treat Res 2004; 119:239–270.
19. Melo JV, Deininger MW. Biology of chronic myelogenous leukemia—signaling pathways of initiation and transformation. Hematol Oncol Clin North Am 2004; 18:545–568, vii-viii.
20. Perrotti D, et al. BCR-ABL suppresses C/EBPalpha expression through inhibitory action of hnRNP E2. Nat Genet 2002; 30:48–58.

21. Skorski T. *BCR/ABL* regulates response to DNA damage: the role in resistance to genotoxic treatment and in genomic instability. Oncogene 2002; 21:8591–8604.
22. Trotta R, et al. *BCR/ABL* activates mdm2 mRNA translation via the La antigen. Cancer Cell 2003; 3:145–160.
23. Neviani P, et al. The tumor suppressor PP2A is functionally inactivated in blast crisis CML through the inhibitory activity of the *BCR/ABL*-regulated SET protein. Cancer Cell 2005; 8:355–368.
24. Donato NJ, et al. *BCR-ABL* independence and LYN kinase overexpression in chronic myelogenous leukemia cells selected for resistance to STI571. Blood 2003; 101:690–698.
25. Ptasznik A, Nakata Y, Kalota A, Emerson SG, Gewirtz AM. Short interfering RNA (siRNA) targeting the Lyn kinase induces apoptosis in primary, and drug-resistant, BCR-ABL1(+) leukemia cells. Nat Med 2004; 10:1187–1189.
26. Donato NJ, et al. Imatinib mesylate resistance through *BCR-ABL* independence in chronic myelogenous leukemia. Cancer Res 2004; 64:672–677.
27. Dai Y, Rahmani M, Corey SJ, Dent P, Grant S. A Bcr/Abl-independent, Lyn-dependent form of imatinib mesylate (STI-571) resistance is associated with altered expression of Bcl-2. J Biol Chem 2004; 279:34,227–34,239.
28. Hu Y, et al. Requirement of Src kinases Lyn, Hck and Fgr for *BCR-ABL1*-induced B-lymphoblastic leukemia but not chronic myeloid leukemia. Nat Genet 2004; 36:453–461.
29. Skorski T, et al. Phosphatidylinositol-3 kinase activity is regulated by *BCR/ABL* and is required for the growth of Philadelphia chromosome-positive cells. Blood 1995; 86:726–736.
30. Carlesso N, Frank DA, Griffin JD. Tyrosyl phosphorylation and DNA binding activity of signal transducers and activators of transcription (STAT) proteins in hematopoietic cell lines transformed by Bcr/Abl. J Exp Med 1996; 183:811–820.
31. Sattler M, et al. Critical role for Gab2 in transformation by *BCR/ABL*. Cancer Cell 2002; 1:479–492.
32. Skorski T, et al. Transformation of hematopoietic cells by *BCR/ABL* requires activation of a PI-3 k/Akt-dependent pathway. Embo J 1997; 16:6151–6161.
33. Vivanco I, Sawyers CL. The phosphatidylinositol 3-kinase AKT pathway in human cancer. Nat Rev Cancer 2002; 2:489–501.
34. Nieborowska-Skorska M, et al. Signal transducer and activator of transcription (STAT)5 activation by *BCR/ABL* is dependent on intact Src homology (SH)3 and SH2 domains of *BCR/ABL* and is required for leukemogenesis. J Exp Med 1999; 189:1229–1242.
35. Ye D, Wolff N, Li L, Zhang S, Ilaria RL Jr. STAT5 signaling is required for the efficient induction and maintenance of CML in mice. Blood 2006.
36. Peters DG, et al. Activity of the farnesyl protein transferase inhibitor SCH66336 against *BCR/ABL*-induced murine leukemia and primary cells from patients with chronic myeloid leukemia. Blood 2001; 97:1404–1412.
37. Sawyers CL, McLaughlin J, Witte ON. Genetic requirement for Ras in the transformation of fibroblasts and hematopoietic cells by the Bcr-Abl oncogene. J Exp Med 1995; 181:307–313.
38. Chu S, Holtz M, Gupta M, Bhatia R. *BCR/ABL* kinase inhibition by imatinib mesylate enhances MAP kinase activity in chronic myelogenous leukemia CD34+ cells. Blood 2004; 103:3167–3174.
39. Notari M, et al. A MAPK/HNRPK pathway controls *BCR/ABL* oncogenic potential by regulating MYC mRNA translation. Blood 2006; 107:2507–2516.
40. Yu C, et al. Pharmacologic mitogen-activated protein/extracellular signal-regulated kinase kinase/mitogen-activated protein kinase inhibitors interact synergistically with STI571 to induce apoptosis in Bcr/Abl-expressing human leukemia cells. Cancer Res 2002; 62:188–199.
41. Dierov JK, Schoppy DW, Carroll M. CML progenitor cells have chromosomal instability and display increased DNA damage at DNA fragile sites. Blood 2005; 106(suppl):1989.
42. Wagner K, et al. Absence of the transcription factor CCAAT enhancer binding protein alpha results in loss of myeloid identity in bcr/abl-induced malignancy. Proc Natl Acad Sci USA 2006; 103:6338–6343.

43. Perrotti D, Marcucci G, Caligiuri MA. Loss of C/EBP alpha and favorable prognosis of acute myeloid leukemias: a biological paradox. J Clin Oncol 2004; 22:582–584.
44. Jones LC, et al. Expression of C/EBPbeta from the C/ebpalpha gene locus is sufficient for normal hematopoiesis in vivo. Blood 2002; 99:2032–2036.
45. Guerzoni C, et al. Inducible activation of C/EBP{beta}, a gene negatively regulated by BCR/ABL, inhibits proliferation and promotes differentiation of BCR/ABL-expressing cells. Blood 2006; 108:1353–1362.
46. Sawyers CL, Callahan W, Witte ON. Dominant negative MYC blocks transformation by ABL oncogenes. Cell 1992; 70:901–910.
47. Skorski T, et al. Antisense oligodeoxynucleotide combination therapy of primary chronic myelogenous leukemia blast crisis in SCID mice. Blood 1996; 88:1005–1012.
48. Xie S, Lin H, Sun T, Arlinghaus, RB. Jak2 is involved in c-Myc induction by Bcr-Abl. Oncogene 2002; 21:7137–7146.
49. Wong KK, et al. A role for c-Abl in c-myc regulation. Oncogene 1995; 10:705–711.
50. Wong KK, et al. v-Abl activates c-myc transcription through the E2F site. Mol Cell Biol 1995; 15:6535–6544.
51. Zou X, Rudchenko S, Wong K, Calame K. Induction of c-myc transcription by the v-Abl tyrosine kinase requires Ras, Raf1, and cyclin-dependent kinases. Genes Dev 1997; 11:654–662.
52. Michelotti EF, Michelotti GA, Aronsohn, AI, Levens, D. Heterogeneous nuclear ribonucleoprotein K is a transcription factor. Mol Cell Biol 1996; 16:2350–2360.
53. Evans JR, et al. Members of the poly (rC) binding protein family stimulate the activity of the c-myc internal ribosome entry segment in vitro and in vivo. Oncogene 2003; 22:8012–8020.
54. Melo JV. The diversity of BCR-ABL fusion proteins and their relationship to leukemia phenotype. Blood 1996; 88:2375–2384.
55. Gribble SM, et al. Genomic imbalances in CML blast crisis: 8q24.12-q24.13 segment identified as a common region of over-representation. Genes Chromosomes Cancer 2003; 37:346–358.
56. Feinstein E, et al. p53 in chronic myelogenous leukemia in acute phase. Proc Natl Acad Sci USA 1991; 88:6293–6297.
57. Honda H, et al. Acquired loss of p53 induces blastic transformation in p210(bcr/abl)-expressing hematopoietic cells: a transgenic study for blast crisis of human CML. Blood 2000; 95:1144–1150.
58. Skorski T, et al. Blastic transformation of p53-deficient bone marrow cells by p210bcr/abl tyrosine kinase. Proc Natl Acad Sci USA 1996; 93:13,137–13,142.
59. Iervolino A, et al. hnRNP A1 nucleocytoplasmic shuttling activity is required for normal myelopoiesis and BCR/ABL leukemogenesis. Mol Cell Biol 2002; 22:2255–2266.
60. Liedtke M, Pandey P, Kumar S, Kharbanda S, Kufe D. Regulation of Bcr-Abl-induced SAP kinase activity and transformation by the SHPTP1 protein tyrosine phosphatase. Oncogene 1998; 17:1889–1892.
61. Chen P, et al. FLT3/ITD mutation signaling includes suppression of SHP-1. J Biol Chem 2005; 280:5361–5369.
62. Wu C, Guan Q, Wang Y, Zhao ZJ, Zhou GW. SHP-1 suppresses cancer cell growth by promoting degradation of JAK kinases. J Cell Biochem 2003; 90:1026–1037.
63. Wu C, Sun M, Liu L, Zhou GW. The function of the protein tyrosine phosphatase SHP-1 in cancer. Gene 2003; 306:1–12.
64. Shet AS, Jahagirdar BN, Verfaillie CM. Chronic myelogenous leukemia: mechanisms underlying disease progression. Leukemia 2002; 16:1402–1411.
65. Skorski T. Oncogenic tyrosine kinases and the DNA-damage response. Nat Rev Cancer 2002; 2:351–360.
66. Deutsch E, et al. BCR-ABL down-regulates the DNA repair protein DNA-PKcs. Blood 2001; 97:2084–2090.
67. Wang H, et al. Efficient rejoining of radiation-induced DNA double-strand breaks in vertebrate cells deficient in genes of the RAD52 epistasis group. Oncogene 2001; 20:2212–2224.

68. Nacht M, et al. Mutations in the p53 and SCID genes cooperate in tumorigenesis. Genes Dev 1996; 10:2055–2066.
69. Sharpless NE, et al. Impaired nonhomologous end-joining provokes soft tissue sarcomas harboring chromosomal translocations, amplifications, and deletions. Mol Cell 2001; 8:1187–1196.
70. Deutsch E, et al. Down-regulation of BRCA1 in *BCR-ABL*-expressing hematopoietic cells. Blood 2003; 101:4583–4588.
71. Jasin M. Homologous repair of DNA damage and tumorigenesis: the BRCA connection. Oncogene 2002; 21:8981–8993.
72. Starita LM, Parvin JD. The multiple nuclear functions of BRCA1: transcription, ubiquitination and DNA repair. Curr Opin Cell Biol 2003; 15:345–350.
73. Slupianek A, et al. *BCR/ABL* regulates mammalian RecA homologs, resulting in drug resistance. Mol Cell 2001; 8:795–806.
74. Shinohara A, Ogawa T. Homologous recombination and the roles of double-strand breaks. Trends Biochem Sci 1995; 20:387–391.
75. Nowicki MO, et al. *BCR/ABL* oncogenic kinase promotes unfaithful repair of the reactive oxygen species-dependent DNA double-strand breaks. Blood 2004; 104:3746–3753.
76. Koptyra M, et al. *BCR/ABL* kinase induces self-mutagenesis via reactive oxygen species to encode imatinib resistance. Blood 2006.
77. Dierov J, Dierova R, Carroll M. *BCR/ABL* translocates to the nucleus and disrupts an ATR-dependent intra-S phase checkpoint. Cancer Cell 2004; 5:275–285.
78. Huntly BJ, Bench A, Green AR. Double jeopardy from a single translocation: deletions of the derivative chromosome 9 in chronic myeloid leukemia. Blood 2003; 102:1160–1168.
79. Brain JM, Goodyer N, Laneuville P. Measurement of genomic instability in preleukemic P190BCR/ABL transgenic mice using inter-simple sequence repeat polymerase chain reaction. Cancer Res 2003; 63:4895–4898.
80. Mori N, et al. Absence of microsatellite instability during the progression of chronic myelocytic leukemia. Leukemia 1997; 11:151–152.
81. Johansson B, Fioretos T, Mitelman F. Cytogenetic and molecular genetic evolution of chronic myeloid leukemia. Acta Haematol 2002; 107:76–94.
82. Sill H, Goldman JM, Cross NC. Homozygous deletions of the p16 tumor-suppressor gene are associated with lymphoid transformation of chronic myeloid leukemia. Blood 1995; 85:2013–2016.
83. Pear WS, et al. Efficient and rapid induction of a chronic myelogenous leukemia-like myeloproliferative disease in mice receiving P210 bcr/abl-transduced bone marrow. Blood 1998; 923780–3792.
84. Zhang DE, et al. Absence of granulocyte colony-stimulating factor signaling and neutrophil development in CCAAT enhancer binding protein alpha-deficient mice. Proc Natl Acad Sci USA 1997; 94:569–574.
85. Ghannam G, et al. The oncogene Nup98-HOXA9 induces gene transcription in myeloid cells. J Biol Chem 2004; 279:866–875.
86. Tanaka T, et al. Dual functions of the AML1/Evi-1 chimeric protein in the mechanism of leukemogenesis in t(3;21) leukemias. Mol Cell Biol 1995; 15:2383–2392.
87. Kantarjian HM, et al. Chronic myelogenous leukemia in blast crisis. Analysis of 242 patients. Am J Med 1987; 83:445–454.
88. Cohen MH, Johnson JR, Pazdur R. U.S. Food and Drug Administration Drug Approval Summary: conversion of imatinib mesylate (STI571; Gleevec) tablets from accelerated approval to full approval. Clin Cancer Res 2005; 11:12–19.
89. Asimakopoulos FA, et al. ABL1 methylation is a distinct molecular event associated with clonal evolution of chronic myeloid leukemia. Blood 1999; 94:2452–2460.
90. Wang JY. Regulation of cell death by the Abl tyrosine kinase. Oncogene 2000; 19:5643–5650.
91. Wlodarski P, et al. Role of p53 in hematopoietic recovery after cytotoxic treatment. Blood 1998; 91:2998–3006.
92. Hernandez-Boluda JC., et al. Genomic p16 abnormalities in the progression of chronic myeloid leukemia into blast crisis: a sequential study in 42 patients. Exp Hematol 2003; 31:204–210.

93. Park IK, et al. Bmi-1 is required for maintenance of adult self-renewing haematopoietic stem cells. Nature 2003; 423:302–305.
94. Tao W, Levine AJ. P19(ARF) stabilizes p53 by blocking nucleo-cytoplasmic shuttling of Mdm2. Proc Natl Acad Sci USA 1999; 96:6937–6941.
95. Kuo ML, et al. Arf induces p53-dependent and -independent antiproliferative genes. Cancer Res 2003; 63:1046–1053.
96. Ahuja HG, Jat PS, Foti A, Bar-Eli M, Cline MJ. Abnormalities of the retinoblastoma gene in the pathogenesis of acute leukemia. Blood 1991; 78:3259–3268.
97. Seeling JM, et al. Regulation of beta-catenin signaling by the B56 subunit of protein phosphatase 2A. Science 1999; 283:2089–2091.
98. Hahn WC, Weinberg RA. Modelling the molecular circuitry of cancer. Nat Rev Cancer 2002; 2:331–341.
99. Miething C, et al. The Bcr-Abl mutations T315I and Y253H do not confer a growth advantage in the absence of imatinib. Leukemia 2006; 20:650–657.
100. Muller C, et al. Separation of C/EBPalpha-mediated proliferation arrest and differentiation pathways. Proc Natl Acad Sci USA 1999; 96:7276–7281.

11

Early Intensification of Therapy: The Role of High-Dose Imatinib and Imatinib-Based Combinations

François Guilhot, Géraldine Martineau, Frédéric Millot, and Lydia Roy
Department of Oncology-Hematology and Cell Therapy, Clinical Research Centre, Poitiers, France

INTRODUCTION

Imatinib has been recognized as a major treatment for patients with chronic myelogenous leukemia (CML). Following several phase I and II trials, a large multicenter phase III trial (IRIS trial) was designed to compare imatinib at standard dose (400 mg) with IFN in combination with low dose cytarabine (1). The long-term benefits of this trial are clearly encouraging (2). The overall estimated survival at 60 months was 89%, with a small proportion of patients who had relapsed or progressed. In all 6.3% of patients progressed to accelerated or acute phase, 5.1% lost their major molecular response and 2.5% lost their hematological response.

Thus imatinib is effective in treating CML. However, some patients ultimately relapse with resistant disease. Resistance may develop through several mechanisms, such as point mutations within the tyrosine kinase binding site, gene amplification, clonal evolution, or decreased imatinib bioavailability (3). In addition, despite the high rate of complete cytogenetic response, a minority of patients achieved a complete and durable molecular negativity and most of the patients who stopped imatinib might have relapsed. This suggests that, although imatinib is highly active against a mature CML cell population, it fails, at least at standard dose, to eradicate all residual leukemic cells. There is evidence that CML stem cells are not eliminated by imatinib in vivo with patients in complete cytogenetic response (CCyR) having detectable Ph+ CD34+ cells and long-term culture initiating cells (LTC-ICs) (4,5).

Thus researches are currently in progress to further elucidate the mechanisms of imatinib resistance and to develop strategies that will expand the usefulness of imatinib. Strategies to overcome imatinib resistance that might occur at the standard of 400 mg/day include imatinib-based combination therapies and high dose imatinib. Others involving novel, more potent tyrosine kinase inhibitors or agents aimed at other targets are discussed in Chapters 5, 6, and 9.

HIGH DOSE IMATINIB

Several observations had suggested that higher dosages of imatinib might be more effective. The initial phase I trial showed a clear dose response relationship (6). In this trial, an hematologic response was observed in all patients treated in chronic phase with imatinib at doses ≥ 140 mg/day. A complete hematologic response was recorded in 98% of patients (53 out of 54) treated at ≥ 300 mg/day, whereas complete responses occurred in only 38% of patients treated with doses lower than 300 mg. Pharmacokinetic studies revealed that above 300 mg plasma levels equivalent to the effective in vitro level (1 μM) were achieved. At dose 400 mg the recommended standard for CML in chronic phase peak levels at steady state were 4.6 μM and through levels at steady state were 2.13 μM, with a half-life of 19.3 hours. In a phase II study, which enrolled 235 patients in accelerated phase, a relationship was also detected between dose and response (7). Patients in accelerated phase treated with 600 mg imatinib daily had higher response rates, improved 12 months survival, and longer responses compared to patients treated with 400 mg daily. In a group of 54 patients with Ph+ CML in chronic phase and with hematological or cytogenetic resistance or relapse on imatinib at 400 mg, a dose increase to 600 mg or 800 mg resulted in subsequent response (8). Complete hematologic response was obtained in 65% of patients, and 56% of those with cytogenetic resistance or relapse achieved MCyR. Thus, higher doses of imatinib can recapture hematologic and cytogenetic responses after failure to standard dose. Based on these preliminary results and observations, higher doses of imatinib were recently investigated. High dose imatinib can be considered as a reasonable option, since most of these studies have shown no maximum tolerated dose and no increase in non-hematological toxicity at doses up to 1000 mg/day. Higher doses of imatinib have been investigated in chronic phase in patients previously treated or in patients who were naïve.

A first study included 37 patients with CML in chronic phase, those who had failed IFN-α and subsequently received imatinib 800 mg daily (9). Overall, 89% of the patients achieved a complete cytogenetic response, in comparison to 48% with standard dose imatinib in a historical control, having a similar patient population. The levels of BCR-ABL/ABL decreased rapidly: by nine months of therapy, over half of the patients had reached levels <0.045%. These levels correspond roughly to a major molecular response. At the last followup, 50% of the patients had reached undetectable BCR-ABL levels by quantitative PCR, confirmed by nested PCR. These molecular response rates are unprecedented with any other medical therapy for CML, including standard dose imatinib. Although the long-term implications of these major and complete molecular remissions are unknown, early data suggest that they correlate with a highly durable complete cytogenetic remission.

A second study investigated the efficacy and toxicity of high dose (HD) imatinib (800 mg daily) in a group of 208 newly diagnosed chronic phase CML patients (10,11).

These data were compared with a historical cohort of 50 patients with newly diagnosed CML treated at the same institution in the preceding year but at the standard dose (SD) of 400 mg and updated at the American Society of Clinical Oncology (ASCO) 42nd Annual Meeting (11).

Cytogenetic and molecular responses were possible to be evaluated in 255 patients ($N = 49$ at SD, 206 at HD) and 248 patients ($N = 46$ at SD, 202 at HD), respectively. In HD group, Sokal risk classification was good in 63%, intermediate in 27%, and poor in 10% of patients. There were no differences in pretreatment characteristics between two groups. The median age was 48 years in both groups. Median followup is 58 months for SD and 34 months for HD group. Patients treated with HD had a higher rate of complete cytogenetic responses (91% vs. 78% with SD, $p = 0.03$) and these occurred earlier, with 76% achieving this response by six months of the therapy versus 51% with SD ($p = 0.0004$). The cumulative incidence of major molecular response was significantly better in HD

TABLE 1 Efficacy of High Dose Gleevec/Glivec in Phase II Trials Compared with the Standard Dose of 400 mg

		IRIS trial (STI571 0106) 400 mg $n = 553$ (%)	400 mg $n = 50$ (8,11) (%)	800 mg $n = 208$ (10,11) (%)	600 mg $n = 75$ (12) (%)
CCyR	Overall	82	78	91	NA
	6 months	52	51	76	80
	12 months	68	75	95	89
MMR	6 months	21	5	38	31
	12 months	39	19	48	45
	24 months	55	60	72	65
4 log reduction	12 months				13
	24 months				29
PCR undetectable		4	29	37	NA

Abbreviations: CCyR, complete cytogenetic response; MMR, major molecular response.

group ($p < 0.05$), and this response was also observed earlier in HD group: at 12 months 48% in HD and 19% in SD group had achieved this response ($p = 0.0001$). At 24 months, 46/123 (37%) patients who can be evaluated with HD versus 9/31 (29%) of patients in SD group achieved complete molecular remission.

These data are summarized in Table 1 and compared with the results obtained with 400 mg in the IRIS trial.

These data consistently suggest that it is possible that in patients with newly diagnosed CML, the use of 800 mg imatinib as starting dose might have a better efficacy than the standard 400 mg dose. Cortes et al. further reported that treatment with high dose imatinib (800 mg) was the most significant factor associated with an increased probability of achieving a molecular response, particularly at early time points (12 months).

The Australian group conducted a phase II trial (TIDEL), in de novo CML patients, using imatinib 600 mg initially, increasing to 800 mg in case of insufficient response: (*i*) nonhematologic response after three months of treatment, (*ii*) no MCyR at six months, (*iii*) no CCyR at nine months, or (*iv*) <4 log reduction in BCR-ABL at 12 months (12). Out of the 101 patients included in the trial, 81 were assessable for the 24 months molecular response. By 12 months 89%, 45%, and 13% had achieved CCyR, ≥3 log, and ≥4 log reductions, respectively. By 24 months 92%, 65%, and 29% achieved these response levels. It was concluded that a more dose intense approach to the treatment of newly diagnosed CML patients achieved a better rate of major molecular response than lower doses, and that maintenance of dose intensity in the first six months of therapy was predictive of molecular response.

The GIMEMA (Italian) group conducted a phase II trial of imatinib 800 mg in intermediate Sokal risk in the early chronic phase of CML (13). Out the 44 patients who completed six months of the treatment, the CHR rate was 100%, and the MCyR and CCyR rates were 90% and 81%, respectively. The major molecular response rate at six months was 56%. A multinational working group (Italy, Nordic Countries, Turkey, and Israel), within the frame of Leukemia Net is exploring 400 mg versus 800 mg in high Sokal risk patients. At the present time, 80 patients have been enrolled but results are pending.

An interim analysis of a multicenter phase II trial (the RIGHT trial) has been recently presented (14).

TABLE 2 Response to High Dose Imatinib—Interim Analysis of the
RIGHT Trial

	N°/N° Evaluable (%) at	
Response	6 Mo (n = 89)	12 Mo (n = 39)
CHR	83 (94)	39 (100)
Cytogenetic		
Complete	NA[a]	33 (85)
Partial	NA[a]	3 (8)
Molecular		
≥3 log ⇓	49 (55)[b]	25 (64)
Undetectable	39 (44)[b]	17 (44)

[a]Not available.
[b]Two patients have missing data.
Abbreviation: CHR, complete hematologic response.

This phase II trial included 115 patients in 29 institutions. These patients received 800 mg imatinib/day and treatment dose was adjusted for ≥3 toxicity grades. The primary endpoint of the trial is molecular response at the first year. Sokal classification was predominantly low (73.1%) or intermediate (17.3%). Peripheral blood PCR and FISH were measured every three months in a central laboratory. Table 2 described the interim analysis of this trial with a high rate of CCyR at 12 months (85%) and a high rate of major molecular response at six months (55%) and 12 months (64%).

IMATINIB IN COMBINATION

In order to obtain a higher rate of cytogenetic response and to overcome resistances, new strategies using combination of cytotoxic drugs with imatinib have emerged. Drugs, which are currently tested, are those that have been selected in the past for their high antileukemic activity. Interferon, pegylated or nonpegylated forms, and cytarabine at various dosages are being actively tested. The conjugation of a 40kDa branched polyethylene glycol molecule to interferonα2a (Peg-IFNα2a) results in the formation of a novel IFN with properties including sustained absorption and a prolonged half life, allowing for a once weekly dosing regimen. Thus this new compound could be better tolerated in CML patients. An open label trial included 144 patients comparing subcutaneous single-agent Peg-IFNα2a 450 µg once weekly with regular IFNα2a, 9 MU/day. After 12 months major cytogenetic response, complete cytogenetic response, as well as hematologic response were significantly better with Peg-IFNα2a as compared with regular IFNα2a, 35% and 18% ($p = 0.0016$), 15% and 7%, 66% and 41% (0.0008) respectively (15). These results suggest that pegylated interferon is not only a more convenient alternative to regular interferon, but also possibly more effective.

The French CML group performed a phase II study of imatinib at a daily fixed dose of 400 mg in combination with Ara-C at 20 mg/m^2 on days 14 to 28 with cycles repeated every 28 days. Thirty patients with previously untreated CML in chronic phase within six months of diagnosis were enrolled (16). Adverse events were frequently observed with grade 3 or grade 4 hematologic toxicities and nonhematologic toxicities in 53% ($n = 16$) and in 27% ($n = 8$) of patients, respectively. The cumulative incidence of CCyR at 12 months was 83% and at six months 100% of the patients achieved CHR (Table 3).

TABLE 3 Hematologic and Cytogenetic Responses Obtained with the Combination Imatinib and Cytarabine

	3 mo	6 mo	9 mo	12 mo
N° of patients at risk	30	30	30	30
Complete hematologic	30[a]	30	30	29
response (95% CI)	100% (88–100)	100% (88–100)	100% (88–100)	97% (83–100)
Cytogenetic response				
Major	21	22	23	25
	70% (51–85)	73% (54–88)	77% (58–90)	83% (65–94)
Complete	7	17	16	21
	23% (10–42)	57% (37–75)	53% (34–72)	70% (51–85)
Partial	14	5	7	4
	47 (28–66)	17% (10–42)	23% (10–42)	13% (4–31)
Minor	2	3	2	2
Failure	2	2	1	1
Not assessable[b]	5	3	4	2

[a]Among the 30 patients, 2 were already in CHR at study treatment.
[b]Not assessable patients: 12 for technical failure; 2 not done.

An exploratory study was conducted in order to investigate the effects of a standard 400 mg daily imatinib dose and a variable pegylated interferon (PegIFN) dose (50 μg/wk, 100 μg/wk, and 150 μg/wk) (17). The criteria for dose adjustment were designed so as to ensure the delivery of the imatinib dose and to protect life quality. There were 76 patients with previously untreated Ph positive CML enrolled in the study. There were three patients who discontinued imatinib and 45 patients who discontinued PegIFN. The severity of adverse events increased with increasing PegIFN dose. The planned imatinib dose could be administered to the patients who were assigned to receive 50 μg/wk or 100 μg/wk PegIFN, but not to those who were assigned to receive 150 μg/wk. The median administered dose of PegIFN ranged between 32 μg/wk and 36 μg/wk. In this group of patients, 70% achieved CCyR and 83% MCyR. The *BCR-ABL* transcript was reduced by at least 3 logs in 68% of CCyR patients (Table 4). These two phase II trials were essential for the design of the current large phase III trials.

Preliminary results of a randomized trial of high dose imatinib with or without PEG-IFN and GM-CSF frontline therapy were recently presented. Patients with previously untreated CP CML started treatment with imatinib 800 mg daily and randomized after six months of therapy to either continue high dose imatinib alone or add PEG-IFN 0.5 mcg/kg/week and GM-CSF 125 mg/m² three times

TABLE 4 Cytogenetic Responses with the Combination Imatinib (400 mg daily) + PegIFN (Percentage)

	TOTAL (n = 76)		50 μg/week (n = 27)		100 μg/week (n = 18)		150 μg/week (n = 31)	
	CCyR	MCyR	CCyR	MCyR	CCyR	MCyR	CCyR	MCyR
3 months	29	61	22	59	33	67	32	58
6 months	46	67	44	78	50	61	45	61
9 months	54	63	48	63	56	61	58	65
12 months	68	79	74	93	67	78	65	68
Overall	70	83	78	93	67	78	65	77

TABLE 5 Patient Characteristics and Response (Intention to Treat)

	N°/N° Evaluable (%)			
	Overall	IM[a] alone	IM + PEG-IFN + GM	p Value
Median age (range), y	48 (19–73)	46 (19–73)	50 (19–73)	0.12
Sokal (% low/int/high)	71/20/9	63/25/12	79/16/5	0.17
CCyR Overall	73/84 (87)	40/45 (89)	33/39 (85)	0.74
at 12 mo	44/49 (90)	27/31(87)	17/18 (94)	0.63
12 mo BCR-ABL/ABL				
<0.05%	20/49 (41)	10/31(32)	10/18 (55)	0.13
Undetectable	5/49 (10)	3/31(10)	2/18 (11)	1.0
Median (range)	0.1 (0–79.3)	0.12 (0–79.3)	0.04 (0–21.9)	0.51

[a]IM, imatinib.
Abbreviation: CCyR, complete cytogenetic response.

weekly (18). Patients were monitored with real time PCR and cytogenetics every three months for the first year and every six months thereafter. Ninety-four patients have been registered: 49 randomized to imatinib alone and 45 to IM + PEG–IFN + GM. 70 (75%) have been followed for at least six months and 49 (52%) for 12 months (first interim analysis was done when 30 patients were in a position to be evaluated at 12 months). Ten patients randomized to PEG-IFN did not start therapy (two refused, two physician's decision, six off study before six months because of noncompliance $n = 3$, melanoma $n = 1$, financial reasons $n = 1$, or progressive disease $n = 1$). There is a trend for improved response after 12 months with the combination (Table 5). Toxicity with high-dose imatinib was similar to previous reports. The most common grade ≥ 3 toxicity associated with PEG-IFN in the 26 patients reported included fatigue ($n = 7$, 27%), rash ($n = 5$, 19%), depression ($n = 3$, 11%), and headache ($n = 2$, 7%). Twelve patients have required dose reductions of PEG-IFN and three of them (13%) permanently discontinued it. The actual median (range) dose of IM at 12 months was 800 mg (600–800 mg) for IM alone and 800 mg of PEG-IM. It was concluded that the combination of imatinib and PEG- IFN as done here was associated with acceptable toxicity profile.

Based on these preliminary results using combination therapies as well as in vitro data suggesting synergistic or additive effect of imatinib with other agents (19), several national groups are currently conducting trials, exploring various dosages of imatinib (400 mg, 600 mg, and 800 mg) and combination therapies with cytarabine or IFN-α. The U.K. and U.S. groups are exploring a comparison between 400 and 800 mg. In addition, two groups are conducting, in parallel, large phase III trials, exploring dosage of imatinib as well as combination therapies. In July 2002, the German CML-study group activated a four arm randomized controlled trial comparing imatinib 400 mg with imatinib plus IFN-α, imatinib plus cytarabine and imatinib after IFN-α failure. In this trial, high risk patients are randomly assigned to primary imatinib-based therapies including a treatment arm with 800 mg daily (20). A recent evaluation was based on 416 patients with 12 months of followup. Of the 335 patients with cytogenetic evaluation, 63% achieved MCyR and 53% CCyR. The number of patients who progressed each year was very low and 27% of patient achieved a major molecular response. However, an analysis of outcome for the individual treatment groups is not yet available.

In September 2003, the French CML study group started a similar phase III trial (21). The experimental arms are IM 400 mg daily in combination with

Peg-IFN-2a (Peg-IFN2a, 90 μg weekly) or IM 400 mg daily in combination with Ara-C, (20 mg/m^2/day, days 15–28 of 28-day cycles) or IM 600 mg daily. The reference arm is IM 400 mg daily. A first evaluation based on 315 patients with a median time of observation of 12 months demonstrated the feasibility of combination therapies with CHR rate of 82% at three months. Cytogenetic data were available from 154 patients. At six months, 135 patients (87%) achieved a MCyR, being complete in 105 patients (68%). A substantial number of patients experienced grade three-fourth hematological as well as nonhematological toxicities. Similarly, analysis of outcome by treatment group is forthcoming. These studies will be very valuable in establishing the role of high dose imatinib and imatinib-based combinations in the management of CML.

CONCLUSION

Although resistance to imatinib develops most frequently in patients in advanced phase, this event may occur in chronic phase patients. Preliminary results obtained with high dose imatinib as well as with combination therapies are promising. Upfront high dose imatinib achieves higher rate of cytogenetic response and also molecular response. In addition, maintenance of dose intensity within the first six months seems predictive of molecular response. However, the maximum initial dose and escalation schedule remains to be determined. High dose of imatinib may also be used in order to recapture responses in patients who fail or have suboptimal response to standard dose imatinib. A recent report suggested that dose increase up to 1200 mg daily was well tolerated and effective in a group of four patients who underwent a second CcyR (22). Combination therapies are promising with drugs known to be powerful in CML like IFN and Cytarabine. However, numerous other combinations could be tested and new agents are currently under assessment (23,24).

REFERENCES

1. O'Brien S, Guilhot F, Larson RA, et al. The IRIS study: International Randomized Study of Interferon and low dose cytarabine versus STI571 (Imatinib mesylate) in patients with newly diagnosed chronic phase Chronic Myeloid Leukemia. N Engl J Med 2003; 348(11): 994–1004.
2. Guilhot FG, Larson RA, O'Brien SG, et al., on behalf of IRIS Study Group. Long-term benefits of Imatinib for patients newly diagnosed with chronic myelogenous leukaemia in chronic phase: the 5-year update from the IRIS study. Haematologica 2006; 91(s1): 466a.
3. Hochhaus A, Kreil S, Corbin AS, et al. Molecular and chromosomal mechanisms of resistance to imatinib (STI571) therapy. Leukemia 2002; 16(11):2190–2196.
4. Elrick LJ, Jorgensen HG, Mountford JC, et al. Punish the parent not the progeny. Blood 2005; 105(5):1862–1866.
5. Sorel N, Bonnet ML, Guillier M, et al. Evidence of ABL-kinase domain mutations in highly purified primitives populations of patients with chronic myelogenous leukaemia. Biochem Biophys Res Commun 2004; 323(3):728–730.
6. Druker BJ, Talpaz M, Resta DJ, et al. Efficacy and safety of a specific inhibitor of the BCR-ABL tyrosine kinase in chronic myeloid leukemia. N Engl J Med 2001; 344(14): 1031–1037.
7. Talpaz M, Silver RT, Druker BJ, et al. Imatinib induces durable hematologic and cytogenetic responses in patients with accelerated phase chronic myeloid leukemia: results of a phase 2 study. Blood 2002; 99(6):1928–1937.

8. Kantarjian H, Talpaz M, O'Brien S, et al. Dose escalation of imatinib mesylate can overcome resistance to standard-dose therapy in patients with chronic myelogenous leukaemia. Blood 2003; 101(2):473–475.

9. Cortes J, Giles F, O'Brien S, et al. Result of high-dose imatinib mesylate in patients with Philadelphia chromosome-positive chronic myeloid leukemia after failure of interferon-alpha. Blood 2003; 102(1):83–86.

10. Kantarjian H, Talpaz M, O'Brien S, et al. High-dose imatinib mesylate therapy in newly diagnosed Philadelphia chromosome-positive chronic phase chronic myeloid leukemia. Blood 2004; 103(8):2873–2878.

11. Aoki E, Kantarjian H, O'Brien S, et al. High-dose imatinib mesylate treatment in patients with untreated early chronic phase (CP) chronic myeloid leukaemia (CML): 2.5-year follow up. J CO 2006; 24(18S) Part I of II:6535a.

12. Hughes T, Branford S, Reynolds J, et al. Maintenance of Imatinib dose intensity in the first six months of therapy for newly diagnosed patients with CML is predictive of molecular response, independent of the ability to increase dose at a later point. Blood 2005; 106(suppl 1):164a.

13. Rosti G, Martinelli G, Castagnetti F, et al. Imatinib 800 mg: preliminary results of a phase II trial of the GIMEMA CML working party in intermediate Sokal risk patients and status-of-the-art of an ongoing multinational, prospective randomized trial of imatinib standard dose (400 mg daily) vs high dose (800 mg daily) in high Sokal risk patients. Blood 2005; 106(suppl 1):1098a.

14. Cortes J, Giles F, Salvado AJ, et al. Interim analysis of a multicenter trial of High Dose (HD) Imatinib in newly diagnosed early Chronic Phase (CP) Patients with Chronic Myeloid Leukemia (CML). Blood 2005; 106(suppl 1):1085a.

15. Lipton JH, Khoroshko ND, Golenkov AK, et al. The Pegasys CML Study Group. Two-year survival data from a randomized study of peginterferon alfa-2a(40KD) vs interferon alfa -2a in patients with chronic phase chronic myelogenous leukemia. Blood 2003; 102(suppl 1):3363a.

16. Gardembas M, Rousselot P, Tulliez M, et al. Results of a prospective phase 2 study combining imatinib mesylate and cytarabine for the treatment of Philadelphia-positive patients with chronic myelogenous leukemia in chronic phase. Blood 2003; 102(13):4298–4305.

17. Baccarani M, Martinelli G, Rosti G, et al. Imatinib and pegylated human recombinant interferon-α2b in early chronic-phase chronic myeloid leukemia. Blood 2004; 104(13):4245–4251.

18. Cortes J, Talpaz M, O'Brien S, et al. A randomized trial of high-dose (HD) Imatinib Mesylate (IM) with or without Peg-Interferon (PEG-IFN) and GM-CSF as frontline therapy for patients with Chronic Myeloid Leukemia (CML) in early Chronic Phase (CP). Blood 2005; 106(suppl 1):1084a.

19. Kano Y, Akutsu M, Tsunoda S, et al. In vitro cytotoxic effects of a tyrosine kinase inhibitor STI571 in combination with commonly used antileukemic agents. Blood 2001; 97(7):1999–2007.

20. Berger U, Hochhaus A, Pfirrmann M, et al. Concept, feasibility and results of the randomized comparison of imatinib combination therapies for chronic myeloid leukemia : the german CML-study IV. Blood 2005; 106(suppl 1):1083a.

21. Guerci A, Nicolini F, Maloisel F, et al. Randomized comparison of imatinib with imatinib combination therapies in newly diagnosed chronic myelogenous leukemia patients in chronic phase: design and first interim analysis of a phase III trial from the French CML group. Blood 2005; 106(suppl 1):168a.

22. Piazza RG, Magistroni V, Andreoni F, et al. Imatinib dose increase up to 1200 mg daily can induce new durable complete cytogenetic remissions in relapsed Ph+ chronic myeloid leukemia patients. Leukemia 2005; 19(11):1985–1987.

23. Chuah C, Tipping AJ, Goldman, et al. Zoledronate is active against Imatinib Mesylate-resistant Chronic Myeloid Leukemia cell lines and synergistic/additive when combined with Imatinib Mesylate. Blood 2003; 102(suppl 1):57a.

24. Dai Y, Rahmani M, Pei XY, et al. Bortezomib and flavopiridol interact synergistically to induce apoptosis in chronic myeloid leukaemia cells resistant to imatinib mesylate through both Bcr/Abl-dependent and –independent mechanisms. Blood 2004; 104(2):509–518.

Index

T - #0146 - 111024 - C172 - 229/152/8 - PB - 9780367453305 - Gloss Lamination